ILLUMINATING LOVE
IN THE HOME
Spotlight on Mental Illness

ILLUMINATING LOVE IN THE HOME
Spotlight on Mental Illness

Book Design: Bonnie Chadburm

Book Cover Design: Brian Call

ISBN: 9781732048003

DEDICATION

There could be endless pages of thanks to those who have given love and encouragement. Let's begin with great gratitude to my spouse who has been through this journey too. He has provided for our family with needs and wants both spiritually and temporally. When times were tough the temptation to bail out and quit was not an option. The characteristics of compassion and trust have strengthened us as a couple. He has walked beside me through the hard and good times. His discipline, loyalty, and love will be eternally recognized and remembered.

My large family is close and I have been blessed to be the oldest of ten children. Our parents are full of love for each one of their posterity. They are leaving a great legacy as they lead by example. To this day, it is with heartfelt gratitude to my family for the kind acts that were extended to me as they were caregivers after two hospitalizations that happened over twenty years ago. They have played a role in wrapping me in their arms with safety and trust so I got up and kept going. The core values that were taught in the home when I was a child have carried me through dark times, until the light began to shine again. Now I am living each day in the present with happiness.

To my seven children and those who have married into our family that have blessed us with fifteen plus grandchildren, may you always feel and know of your infinite worth. They know each one of them has a special place in my heart and have brought me happiness beyond words. Their sweetness and hugs keep my world going in such a fun way.

It is with great thanks to the many health professionals, holistic practitioners, spiritual leaders, teachers, business coaches and mentors, that have used their education to instruct me to know a better way.

My overall results and unusual awareness of what I can do to move forward in life has been a gift from God. This story is one that has proved out to be a great taskmaster to learn self-mastery and how to honor the struggles that help you grow. It is my hope that others can find ways to see light through the darkness so you can live with purpose and passion. See the tender mercies and miracles large and small unfold daily!

To those I know, and to those who I will meet, I thank you for making a difference in this beautiful world. Enjoy these golden nuggets to change your lifestyle to live a rich and abundant life of joy!

Testimonials

This book has many hidden treasures, lessons learned, and most importantly, the message of love and hope can be found in your home even under the most trying of circumstances, whatever they may be.

G. Roai. B.

Once I started reading this book I couldn't put it down. It was amazing information and it let me know how a family coped with mental illness.

Alicia L.

As someone living with a family member who struggles with depression, self-harm, and addiction, I have seen first-hand the misery, torment, desolation, and utter despair which accompanies them. I have experienced the sorrow and heartache of watching someone I care about suffer so. The author's courage in sharing her personal story of anguish and pain, then of faith and healing, will bless the lives of all who read it. It has blessed mine. It is an honor and a privilege to have her as a friend.

Carol D.

It was touching to read the short story of a beautiful mother addressing the loss of a son, and in such a tender and loving way. Sharing how important the role of each member of a family truly is. The healing peace that we can come to know after tragedy strikes home. Suicide is a big problem and I have lost dear friends to this unfortunate and devastating problem. I will be sharing what I've learned from this book and bring hope to those in need.

Stacey B.

This book was a beautiful and unexpected answer to my prayers. I have been on both sides of mental illness through out my life. I have been a caretaker and a mental health patient. Many of the perspectives both from the author and her family members really hit home for me. This book is full of information that can help a person who is struggling and their families to bypass a lot of unnecessary frustration because she breaks down the things that worked for her and the things that didn't and why....that alone was super helpful for me because it helped me see what the possible outcome could be and what freedoms I would lose if I made the decision to act out. The other thing that I loved were the action steps. There were many suggestions listed and many of them I had already been doing so it helped me see that I was on the right path.

I also loved that prayer has been a huge part of her healing process as it has been the key to my healing process. Prayer for specific direction is the best advice there is in my opinion.

This book is so inspired!

I recommend anyone who is dealing with any form of mental illness to read this.

Jen S.

10 GIFTS FOR JOY

IN

MIND AND BODY

INTRODUCTION

What is in this book are my experiences and opinions. There are suggestions and action steps that have been proven to be very effective. Patterns and feelings were discovered after recording and tracking daily. Write and see what works for you.

It has been decided to have minimal editing in order to get this information to you now. With what is going on in the world this is the right time to speak up publicly to shed light on ways you can navigate through stress and trauma. This is more important than having each sentence written perfectly. The family contributions have also been kept intact to preserve the intent of the authors. Too many families are going through the types of challenges described in the different scenarios in the book and are at a loss on what to do and how to see light at the end of the dark tunnel. Move forward with faith and hope that things will work out.

If you need medical advice or treatments seek out the help you need from qualified professionals.

THE INFORMATION IN THIS BOOK IS IN ADDITION TO, AND NOT INSTEAD OF BEING MEDICALLY MONITORED.

Who is this book for?

This book is for:

Those with physical, mental, emotional, spiritual, social, and financial concerns that will all be addressed to assist you in finding wholeness and health.

The title of the book Illuminating Love in the Home-Spotlight on Mental Illness was chosen after much thought and prayer. In Webster's dictionary illuminate means to light up, to lighten, to throw light on, and brighten.

The -ing at the end puts us in the present. Assess the situation as it is right now and how you can make the weightier issues that you are dealing with lighter.   It is the present moment that matters when you are in a crisis situation.   Pure and genuine love will provide the energy you will want to have to get through the tough days.

Home will be addressed literally and figuratively. There is the building that you live in called "Home" that you want to have light and love in. When thinking of the mind and brain, it is housed in the body (another home). Home can be community, friends, office, and neighbors and the qualities wanted are love, safety, support, peace, and so on.

By being comfortable in your own skin, the "You", is the most important "Home" you want to master and focus on. Let your goal be to bring illuminating love and light into all these types of homes so they are filled with joy.

Part of the title of the book-Spotlight on Mental Illness could be replaced with other situations where there is a stigma associated with it such as Spotlight on _____ (money problems, bankruptcy, divorce, unemployment, addiction, homelessness, suicide abuse, etc.)

The specifics of my story are there to help you have a reference to stimulate your mind to find your own path and how they correlate to universal truths.

There also is information for caregivers and what they can do and say. Much of the suggestions can be used by anyone no matter what side of the fence you are on.

3 different stages of the illness
1-Green- has unusual behavior according to society-not funny ...yet kind of funny
2-Yellow-much more abnormal behavior -does not make good decisions-requires constant care
3-*Red-unrecognizable and combative-requires immediate medical attention-or life-threatening behavior
*Seek medical attention ASAP

CONTRIBUTIONS FROM

FAMILY PERSPECTIVES

(Short stories interspersed throughout the book -in Italics)

After reading the contributions tears came to my eyes as I realized how those who were there for me and all that they went through. I had no idea. This was eye opening. Illuminating love was increased in our home as we had conversations. This part of the book has great value to help stimulate ways you can talk and open up to each other to become closer.

I appreciate the support by those who have written these contributions. Great thanks go to my brother for the hours and hours of assistance I received for the book to be able to come into print.

CONTRIBUTION- INSIGHTS FROM A FAMILY CAREGIVER
Daughter

My mother asked me to write my perspective of what it was like being raised by a mother diagnosed with bipolar. *I hope that this perspective will give insight to those of you who may be going through similar circumstances and courage to face whatever challenges lay ahead.*

I am the second oldest of my seven siblings. I am currently in my thirties raising four children of my own and now consequently, have an even greater appreciation for my mother, her willingness to sacrifice for our family and her overwhelming perseverance in the face of so much opposition. I am eternally grateful for a mother that did not give up even when at times it must have seemed like her burdens were too much to bare. Because my mother was willing to persevere and keep going even in the midst of adversity, she has not only changed my life but the lives of my children and her posterity.

Upon reflection of my childhood I look back with fondness and admiration for the level of commitment and dedication my parents had for each other and for each of their children. I always felt loved and I knew that my parents wanted to provide me with opportunities that

15

would further my abilities and help me grow. I had what I would consider an idyllic childhood. At a young age, my parents encouraged us to develop our talents. They provided us with many opportunities to enhance our skills. From as early as four years old, my sisters and I were enrolled in ballet, jazz, and tumbling lessons. As we got a little older, at various times, we were also enrolled in other activities including swimming, singing, piano, and art lessons. I remember enjoying the challenge that each opportunity brought.

My mother would often arrange for all of us to perform at local nursing homes to give us experience being in front of people and also be around people less fortunate than ourselves. We also performed at local festivals and school talent shows. Even now it is exhausting for me to think about the amount of effort that must have gone into preparing all of my siblings to sing and dance at different events.

Growing up, my mother was conscientious and hardworking and always set high expectations for herself. She took exceptional effort to make sure that all of us were always dressed appropriately for church and other functions. Our hair was neatly curled and each of our outfits were carefully chosen to match one another. Now that I am a mother, I understand and am awed at the immense effort that was taken to make

*sure we all looked presentable. I am certain
that getting seven children out the door all dressed
and ready to go for church or any other activity
would have been quite the feat for any mother to
achieve. Unfortunately, all the extra
responsibilities and expectations eventually began
to affect my mother's health.*

*During my fifth-grade year, a few months after my
brother was born, our family would experience a
change of events that would require all of us to
simplify and reduce our extra activities. At the
time, I was currently preparing to perform in the
Nutcracker Ballet. Multiple practices per week
were required and my mother would drive me
thirty-five minutes to practice. About half-way
through my rehearsal schedule my mother's health
took a drastic turn for the worse. She experienced
what doctors would term a "psychotic break."*

*Although an exact cause of a psychotic break is
not completely understood it is suspected that a
genetic predisposition in combination with the
right environmental stressors can help lead up to
such an event. At the time, my mother was under a
substantial amount of stress. My father was an
extremely hard-working devoted dad. He was
involved in the family affairs as much as he could
be. Unfortunately, he worked a retail sales job that
required him to work long hours. In addition to his
full-time job, he also managed apartment rentals*

my parents owned. My dad was also, in the process of starting his own side business and was subsequently preparing to launch an advertising campaign to market a massaging mattress that he had developed. My dad's hectic schedule required my mother to often manage the family on her own. Stressful conditions such as these, are possible examples of the kinds of environmental stressors that often times proceed a psychotic break.

Even though these stressful circumstances may have contributed to a psychotic break it is likely that many other factors played a part. In fact, it is impossible to predict exactly what may or may not have happened had circumstances been different. After conversing with my parents over the years, I have observed that shame and guilt can easily manifest themselves when discussing why these events may have occurred. I have even asked myself if there was something that I could have done different to prevent these events from occurring. Even though it may be a natural tendency to try to scrutinize what things could've been done differently, I have learned that is important to remember, as my mother mentions in her book, that blame and shame can delay healing and ought to be avoided as much as possible.

Indeed, the honest truth is that events happen for a reason and we can always choose to let circumstances define who we are or choose to learn from them instead. I myself am more compassionate and understanding of others who struggle with similar circumstances. I have also learned that certain experiences occur in life that are not always in our control no matter how much we wish they were different. That being said, my mother is the perfect example of someone who has been able to learn from her past. Certainly, she has done all that she can do to take responsibility for the things she can change and not look for someone to blame or allow excuses to prevent her from seeking proper help.

At the time of my mother's first psychotic break, I was only ten years old. I was too young to fully understand what was going on. My mother went to stay with my grandma for a few days. I was told my mom was under a lot of stress and she no longer would be able to take me to practices. My sisters and I stayed several days with other family members. Carpools were also arranged for me so that I could finish out the holiday season of the Nutcracker. Even though my mother was only absent for a few short days before returning to care for us, when she returned home, her energy level and motivation to participate in family activities seemed diminished.

Throughout the remainder of the year, lessons and other obligations were reduced. At the time, it was difficult for me to understand why we were not able to do as many activities. I would often ask my parents to begin lessons again but the subject was usually casually dismissed. I began spending more hours playing with my siblings often times oblivious to where my mother was or what she was doing. One blessing that occurred from having to simplify was that I was able to develop better relationships with my siblings. To this day my siblings are my best friends. We love being together and thoroughly enjoy each others company.

Throughout my Jr. high years, our daily life carried on as expected. My mother was often tired and would retreat frequently to her room to sleep. Her withdrawal to her room was most likely caused from fatigue and exhaustion due to endless motherly duties as well as side effects from anti-psychotic medication. My mother also gave birth to my baby sister when I was in eighth grade. Although I'm certain this was a happy event, I'm also sure it brought its own set of additional stress and fatigue. Because my mother was often occupied taking care of the younger siblings, it became necessary for the older siblings to contribute more around the house. As a result, at a young age we were expected to work and take care of ourselves.

Some of our weekly responsibilities included taking turns cooking, babysitting, and helping with other various household chores. I'm sure that at the time I begrudgingly completed the tasks that were assigned and probably would've preferred spending more time playing, but the shift in household responsibilities from my mother to the older children made it possible for myself and all of my siblings to learn valuable life lessons. We were able to learn how to work hard, how to be less selfish, how to care for younger siblings, and how to rely on each other.

Near the end of my Sophomore year, my mother experienced another life-threatening psychotic break. The onset of this episode is not completely known but at the time my mother was also under a lot of stress and was physically in a weakened state after recently recovering from bronchitis. This psychotic episode lasted for several weeks. This time I was old enough to know that my mom was distinctly not herself. Her sentences were disconnected and did not make sense. She would giggle and cry within the same sentence. Her speech was jumbled and difficult to understand. She would jump from one topic to the next within a matter of seconds. It was quite obvious that my mother needed help. Soon after my mother's behavior changes, my father took my mother to be cared for by my grandparents.
Although I was confused by my mother's sudden change in behavior, I did not think that it was something that would be permanent. I thought my mom just needed a break and she would be back to

herself within a few days. I did not think any less of my mom, in fact I thought her actions were more likely the result of her constant concern for us. The Sunday after my mother was taken to be cared for by my grandmother's house, a large number of my extended family members gathered together in prayer and fasting on behalf of my mother. My dad along with a few other family members gave my mother a blessing. My mother was promised that she would be able to receive the help that she needed. My mother did not heal immediately; rather with time, patience, and continued faith, my mother was eventually able to receive the help that she would need for her recovery.

On the night of my Junior Prom, which I did not attend because I was not officially sixteen, a friend took me over to my grandparent's house to see my mother. When I saw my mom, I was shocked and surprised at how quickly she had declined. She looked malnourished and disheveled.

Her hair was stringy and her mouth was white and frothy. Dark circles had formed under her eyes most likely caused from many nights with little sleep. She was lying down on a couch staring at the ceiling. Her eyes darted back and forth and I could hear her softly moaning under her breath. It was clearly the first time that I thought, "What if my mother did not come back to herself?" "What if she was never the same." Even worse, "What if my mother died?"

I left my grandparent's house knowing that in order for my mother to recover she was going to need a miracle. She was going to need God to intervene in her behalf and provide the necessary professional help she needed to recover.

Shortly after my visit, it became clear to my grandparents that they no longer could take care of my mother on their own. They recognized that my mother needed more care than they could offer. Not only was her mental health suffering but her physical health was quickly deteriorating. She was no longer eating, drinking, or sleeping.

Soon after, my mother was taken to receive medical attention at the hospital. Within a few short days, with proper and immediate care and with the help of anti-psychotic medication, my mother was able to make a remarkable come back. This was the answer to prayers that all of us had been patiently waiting for.

After my mother's recovery, my brother and all of my sisters were able to return home under the care and supervision of my mother. Our daily routine returned relatively back to normal. Following my mother's return, I was much more hesitant to ask my mother to come to additional school assemblies or various sports events that I was currently involved with. I recognized that adding more requests would only add expectations and additional stress to her already full plate. I remember wishing that I could tell my parents more about what was going on in my life my challenges, my frustrations, my disappointments. Inopportunely, because of the events that had transpired during this time, I wasn't able to fully express my thoughts and concerns to my mom and dad without the fear that I would cause more stress and possibly additional mental instability. I relied heavily on my sisters and friends for support. I will forever be grateful to all of the neighbors, church leaders, and exceptional friends that stepped up and volunteered to help with rides as well as offer their encouragement and love at this particularly vulnerable time.

After my mother's psychotic episodes, it took several years before my mother was comfortable seeking out professional help. Over time, my mother has become more willing to share her experiences with qualified professionals. Under careful management and supervision from a physician, psychiatrist, counselor, and other various mentors my mother has been able to avoid any relapse to the same degree of intensity that occurred during my high school years. Learning to trust medical recommendations and rely on help has not come all at once. It has taken time to evaluate what information and medical advice works most effectively for her individual needs. Gradually my mother has been able to implement specific interventions and recommendations into her daily routine that have helped her manage bipolar. She has learned to document her sleep patterns and monitor her emotions by writing her activities and feelings in a daily journal. She has learned how to rely on my dad and other family members for feedback about her emotions and her daily communication. She has become more conscientious about setting boundaries. She has learned to set limits and say no. She is more in-tune with her own needs and is willing to allow herself to receive adequate rest.

Over the years, I have been able to witness how my mother has pleasantly surprised her doctor's and counselor's expectations. Despite the stigma that often accompanies mental illness, my mother has been able to not only accept her diagnosis but also use her experiences as learning opportunities to help others. When I was younger my mother kept her feelings to herself. In fact, many of the details of her diagnosis were not explained to me until years after I graduated. Throughout my high school years, my mother would avoid crowds and large groups of people.

The beginning stages of her psychotic breaks manifested themselves during a PTA meeting and a church testimony meeting. Both of these instances occurred in front of large groups of people. As a result, these experiences increased my mother's embarrassment and decreased her desire to speak in front of people. She would avoid school assemblies and sporting events as much as possible. Over the course of several years, with time and patience, my mother has since been able to overcome this fear. I have seen her speak confidently and openly on a number of occasions in front of large audiences. She has used these speaking engagements to teach others about how to find hope, healing, and peace in the midst of adversity.

I have always admired the love and respect that my parents have had for one another. Regardless of the uncertainty and unpredictability of bipolar, my dad has stood faithfully by my mother every step of the way. He has helped and encouraged her to seek out and receive the help that she has needed. He has also allowed her the time and flexibility to take care of her own needs. Together, they have demonstrated to all of our family that through commitment, devotion, and patience we can still be steadfast and loyal to each other even when faced with adversity.
Even though this trial has been challenging for all of our family in his or her own individual way, my family has been able to rally together and, in the process, we have learned valuable lessons

about faith, patience, and the power of prayer. We also have learned that sometimes we must be willing to ask for help and then also be willing to accept it. Most importantly, we have learned that even though adversity may come our way, there is always meaning in our suffering.

In conclusion, I would like to thank my mother for all that she has done for me.
She has sacrificed unselfishly so that my siblings and I could enjoy the life that we have. My mother continues to persevere in spite of her challenges and in the process, she continues to teach all the rest of us even more about faith, endurance, and determination. Because of her challenges my mother has become even more compassionate and empathetic towards those who suffer with similar mental illnesses. As a result, she has undertaken the responsibility to share with others her experience of what it feels like to be surrounded in darkness and yet in the midst of that darkness finding hope and light.

Anyone who has been around my mother for long, has unmistakably observed that she is the quintessential essence of hope, light, and love. She is truly an example of pure love, generosity, and kindness. Her trials have made her stronger and subsequently, allowed her to bless the lives of many people; and so it is with all of us if we are ***willing to have hope, courage, and determination to keep on going.***

Contribution-Family Caregiver- (Brother)

I'm a very private person, and usually do not want to have some of this out there, but because of a kind request from my wonderful sister, I put those feelings aside to share some perspectives through great trials and tribulation. These have turned out to be "a blessing". A knowledge of hope and a brighter illumination of love in a family. We discovered how each member has such an important and valuable role in each others lives. Each individual person brings incomprehensible great worth. I would not be showing gratitude if I were to suppress this and especially when others may find it very useful.
So here goes...

Years ago, in a galaxy not that far away, or in other words...in our younger days...

It was a beautiful spring day, and I had just prepared myself for this track meet that was going on at the High School. It was particularly fun because my sister was also a participant. She was a couple of years older than I. It was fun and exciting to have two family members out there on the track competing. I was developing into a very good athlete and enjoyed sports, and my sister...

LOL ...well, let me continue. It is hard to type when you're laughing this hard.
Here is a little family background that may help you to understand more about my sister.

She was the oldest girl of a family of 10, and I was the oldest boy. It was really nice to be able to draft in my sister's footsteps as she was a 4.0 student, and all the teachers and student body loved her. She practically walked on water. So, when I got over to the high school my freshman year, all I had to do is drop a hint that this was my sister and it was almost always guaranteed an "A". Wahoo! School for me was a breeze. Thank you, Sis!

Seems like everything my sister was involved in, such as modeling, school, dating, church, or whatever it was she was doing was a home run as she knocked it out of the park. She was a smart and attractive perfectionist.
Along with intelligence and beauty she was very responsible, kind, sweet, and meek. A pleasure to be around. Almost too good to be true. Right?

So back to the track meet...

The announcer has just called out over the

microphone... "The winner of the mile...Is.... (and he calls out the name of the first-place winner...and 2nd... and so on until all the runners were in.

"Oh, wait just a minute! Clear the track! Clear the track! We still have another runner! We cannot begin the next race until she finishes...Everybody cheer her on Please!... Big round of applause please... Come on...You can do it... Look at that determination!"

I think that someone should have spoken to her that the record she is shooting for should be a low time, not the highest time on school record. When my sister finally came in on her final lap. The crowd erupted into a roar which was 10 times the energy and excitement that was extended to the first, second and third place winners.

My sister was spectacular in absolutely everything that she did in life and was even spectacular on the track, (even though she was the last person to finish every race all season long). Everybody loved her and was cheering her on.

So, let's travel few years later down the road and...
Boom! The illness came:
So, when the news came that my sister was in trouble and "all hands on deck". The calls went out and we are there to support her through the

problem. At the time I was under the impression that there isn't anything we can't get over but have learned through this "Blessing" and when I say blessing, I mean anything that moves you closer to Christ is a blessing. Not just good things only, sometimes prior to this new information that I had learned, I used to say in my prayers : "
I am thankful for: "All my many blessings" and came to realize after this ordeal, that this blessing would be one of the hardest things I have ever experienced in my life. Watching my sister who had the whole world in her hands and was quickly and decisively taken away from her with this mental illness. The repeated question: What to do? What to do?

And now the rest of the story. ...

My sister mentioned she was sharing what happened in the closet. This is added to give more perspective to this ordeal. We tried to take care of her as best we could and had prepared a room in the back bedroom that was nice and out-of-the-way of the general public so that we could work with her until she got better. She started going from a yellow to red stage and talked about jumping out the window and other serious acts that could cause bodily injury, and other "out of the social norm" behaviors.

We realized that this would not work so we prepared a large walk-in closet. The twin size mattress was put on the floor and a couple more mattresses along the wall. It was at this stage that I realized I didn't recognize my sister.

Where was she? It was my turn to be with her all night and I was very tired, but I was scared for her as well. I noticed that she didn't sleep for days on end, and this is a huge problem for caregivers. Thank goodness for large family and taking turns.

After getting the walls lined with mattresses, I instructed her that she can do whatever she wants, but nobody is going in or out of this room until she comes back (mentally). I said to myself that I would be there for my sister and I was more concerned about outside forces getting in and possibly taking over my sister. I was literally a Guardian at the door.

Earlier in the week. My sister had spent some time in the care of my grandmother. I went to raise my hand in preparation of casting out spirits, and my grandmother grabbed my arm and said that is not appropriate at this time. I internally wrestled with this for a while after, but soon learned of the wisdom in my grandmother's action. There is a difference of mental illness and the other, although sometimes this can happen (from my vantage point, of course)

We came up with a measuring system to help us identify and discuss the different stages.

<u>3 different stages of the illness</u>
1-Green- has unusual behavior according to society-not funny ...yet kind of funny
2-Yellow-much more abnormal behavior -does not make good decisions-requires constant care
3-*Red-unrecognizable and combative-requires immediate medical attention-or life-threatening behavior *Seek medical attention ASAP.
Some Triggers:
Sleep, Food-(or lack of it) Nutrition, & Stress

After much tribulation and long-suffering, we sought out professional and medical help and were able to find great success.
It has been a trial of fire, but a wonderful blessing as we watch this beautiful young lady that struggled through mental illness and come out the other side. After these trials, I have noticed my sister is a stronger, better, confident mother, mentor, successful business woman, and now author, and continues to amaze all, including the medical profession. They have commented on how she is able to successfully manage her life and problems with solutions and is a beacon to those around her.
*Good job, sis... love you ...**Bro***

CHAPTER 1

THE PRICELESS GIFT OF YOU

The priceless gift of you, starts the day you were born. If you have parents you can take the opportunity to find out the specifics. Do you wonder why this information would be helpful? Even when the circumstance is less than ideal you realize you are alive, a survivor, and made it this far and will keep going. You are ready for the good and the bad to experience all of life. When you know about your name research shows this knowledge can get you through stress. Problems at birth often carry into life and clues of generations can be traced back. This is insightful when trying to make connections to recognize patterns in order to have possible solutions.

What I discovered has been a treasure to me. With some persistence I was able to have both parents share. It is amazing how each little baby wants to write their own story. From day one it was decided that my first grand appearance was going to be different.

I was born in the day when fathers were left in the waiting room much to the dismay of my Dad. He always wanted to be involved in the birth and in my case his wish was granted. Mom was feeling very uncomfortable in the labor room and Dad got a sneak peek of two legs that were black as coal. In his words this was a shocking sight, and when the message was relayed to my young Mother she began to cry. These tears were not because of pain but of fear. Fear of what was yet to be. What would happen to her baby?

That was the beginning of me doing things the opposite way of most people and having things work out. After the nurses were summoned and Mom was taken to the delivery room, one hour turned into two, then three, four, and almost five with two dark legs hanging out. Interns were called to watch the birth and learn. The regular doctor was in need of assistance because of his hand being cut after being bit by a dog. This turned out to be good because Mom had heard things about him she did not like, so having a different person do the delivery was totally fine with her.

Evidently quite a medical crowd was gathered in the room and it came as a surprise to Mom when her second child was born and there was just a handful of people for a normal delivery. It was much later she came to understand the nature of my birth and what a blessing it was that she had a healthy baby.

Dad was born breech at home and the doctor worked and worked on him to bring him to life. Grandma would talk of this horror and so when the experience was turning out to be similar this created more fear in their hearts.

Drops of sweat were pouring off the doctor's face as he tried and tried to get the rest of my body born. When I heard this part of the story I suspect I was struggling to come into mortality. It's amazing to me how my Mom could go through so much and still to this day has said nothing to how much pain she was in. Perhaps it was a blessing for Dad to not be a witness to that part. She's a wonderful woman to bring ten lives into this world.

What she does talk about is the shock and her unhappiness that the doctor's first word when I was being born was a swear word. This poor language was a far cry from what she wanted her sweet new baby angel to hear first. Throughout life my parents set a high standard by living the values they taught and I never heard inappropriate language or fighting all the years I was raised. That's a miracle in and of itself.

Needless to say, hour after hour, Father was pacing in the room. Waiting and waiting to hear what was going on and know the ones he loved were safe. Dad said when I was finally placed in his arms it was like the bright sun coming out after a long dark night.

What resonates in this story are the characteristics that developed to help me navigate through all kinds of stress was to know light follows darkness. Joy follows labor. Example means more than shallow words. Pain and hurt are worth the struggle to have a reward. Each one writes their own story. In the end things work out. People do their best while they are learning. Most of all, love triumphs.

Looking back some of the qualities that I am known for are the same as my parents. Unless you intentionally set out and want to be different you most likely will follow the pattern you were taught from the moment you were born. Day one is the start of your foundation that each one of us is unique, different, and priceless. Sometimes your physical and mental challenges lead back to this day along with the successes.

In the pages ahead thought pattern management will be brought up in how to heal from the past with the subconscious mind working for you. Sometimes birth experiences are used to promote healing. This knowledge was very helpful in what I have been able to do and function at such a high level with a mental illness diagnosis that manifested in my thirties. I am a miracle and grateful to have this blessing to live a rich full life. Ultimately, we are God's creations and his purpose is for each one of us to have peace, and joy!

Contributions in this book have been made from others from their point of view as to what they observed when dealing with me receiving a mental illness bipolar diagnosis. If the person was helping me saw me in a psychotic state the words of what I expressed was mixed up with what happened in the past and current reality. Some of the thoughts and feelings had been pushed down deep into silence and the words were coming out along with things that I thought would happen that were out of reality but very real to me.

It would be extremely difficult for a bystander to be able to decipher the difference between what was fact and fiction. One thing I have come to realize is how many people have wanted to help me over the years that were confused as to how. Vocalize and teach others how they can support and serve you and accept their best of what they can do. Let your feelings not be hurt if the answer is "No" and what help you receive is different than what you had in mind. If you are a caregiver your influence will be much more effective if you keep what you would say to a minimum while their mind is scattered until your loved has received medical attention and stabilized. Be open and honest with what you are doing as much as possible. One thing I remember is when supplements were put in my drinks or overhearing discussions about me led to mistrust. Cooperation will be more likely when you can be upfront because lying and holding back will be sensed.

My story can give you additional insights as to what might come up in order to assist you in being prepared to navigate the possible decisions you may be called on to make. Today I am able to say mental illness has been a gift to me and with time may this be the same for you.

We developed this communication formula to discuss condition in order to know what kind of help was needed. By asking what stage: green, yellow, or red helped in determining actions more quickly.

3 different stages of the illness
1-Green- has unusual behavior according to society-not funny ...yet kind of funny
2-Yellow-much more abnormal behavior -does not make good decisions-requires constant care
3-*Red-unrecognizable and combative-requires immediate medical attention-or life-threatening behavior
*Seek medical attention ASAP.

If you are coping with this now or working with someone who is suffering you know how taxing and stressful mental illness is. It is hoped what knowledge you gather from these perspectives will give understanding of where one person is coming from. Have a synergistic approach that puts ALL parties on a path of hope and healing. There is a trickle down effect that touches each life in a unique way when you face these types of challenges. The contributions in the book gives understanding to that.

It is critical to recognize this for the caregiver to stay strong and not become a casualty of having to be cared for too. You'll be serving your loved one best by taking care of yourself.

When I know there is a lot of needless suffering and silence going on, it is my hope that at least ONE person and possibly more will be helped by this book. If that ends up to be the case, then this labor of love to write this will be worth it.

By speaking up about my own journey of living life to the fullest with a bipolar diagnosis has required being willing to ask and receive help. In order to maintain independence it became necessary to be patient. Give yourself permission to have the space and time to grow. Let your own ideas be stimulated in order for you to seek the answers that will bless you individually.

There is a process to healing!

When one person suffers, then often the caregivers suffer alongside you and is impacted by the illness in a different way. The reality is the solution will be about PURE LOVE and moving forward with courage and compassion unitedly as a team. This is the goal.

Speaking openly on what is commonly left unsaid about mental illness and the challenges and afflictions that come can be freeing. Even though some of the specifics of what is shared here happened long ago there are individuals going through this in their home right now that are at a loss. This is one of the main reasons for sharing.

 If all that is heard is successes and the happy stuff and the problems are glossed over you may find out later you have negative thoughts brewing that will manifest later. As much as you would like the struggles to go poof and instantly disappear this is not likely. Choose to dwell in optimism as you stay real with what you are facing.

Sometimes you hear of a person talking about how good a person has life, or it can be just the opposite where they share one trial after another. The competition in conversations can be who has it the worst or who has it the best. Comparing the good and bad times to what someone else has is a dream killer and a huge trap.

When the suffering is so intense it is vital to use blocks of time that are small. Find peace by accepting and knowing what is worth the effort to change. Progress a day, an hour, a minute, or in moments when needed. Time is a gift! Each day you can learn how to choose to open this gift and how your hours in mortality will be spent to serve others. When I was in deep torture of the mind this became crucial. One tip that has come in handy is to stop taking things personal and remember when the illness is talking and acting out. For the one who goes into recovery this will help you too. This is a nasty no fun illness and sometimes the hard decisions of treatment need to happen so life can be easier in the long run.

Putting all parties into a safe place could be to clarify what you will and will not talk about. Let your focus be on the problem to identify solutions instead of character assassinations. Stay uplifting and calm in your words and discuss the things that are within your realm to change. If someone chooses to take something to heart let it stay their problem and not yours. Realize what the person is going through is about them instead of you.

Caregivers wait and make sure the person that is hurting is being heard and understood! Be free of distraction and look them in the eye. If you are on the receiving end of the conversation LISTEN

FIRST. This means STOP yourself from prematurely interjecting with the council of: "Let me tell you…sell you…advise you…there is only one way… I told you so..." plus more. Once you think you "Get it" put these comments on the back burner until you have made a solid connection and use restraint and caution when offering YOUR solution. If possible trust them to be able to figure things out.

It's amazing how much more you will find when you stay silent and take a long pause. Commonly the person will start talking again. Use words that instill principles of trust, love, and confidence. By remembering that you can go through hard things and believe in yourself will keep you going and the parties involved will have some relief so the burdens stay lighter.

Trials as well as the victories have value. Being able say what works can save another person time, and perhaps even their life. Statistics are extremely high for those who have mental illness to choose to end their own existence. Suicide leaves a trail of tears. Get on top of things by seeking knowledge and people that can assist you to implement what you learn so you can live peacefully with those around you. Stay accountable.

Let the joyous times far exceed the dark times by CHOOSING the thoughts you are going to DWELL on. When someone is in a bottomless pit it is a great reward to see them rising to the top.

Please, please, please, reach out and connect if you feel you are in a fragile state of mind. Choose to keep going!

There is a story called the cyper in the snow that illustrates the state of mind and a dream that was very common for me where I would disappear and be found frozen to death. It was easy to be in a crowded room and feel alone. Being quiet and staying unseen was where the dangerous comfort was. What has been discovered is how critical it was to reach out and try to connect. Uncomfortable was the beginning solution to inner peace and health.

As you read my story you will find how essential it became to love myself. In the Bible it says Love thy neighbor AS thyself. Sometimes I wonder how many are remembering what comes after AS. Loving yourself and others is a great gift to the world. In fact, the most important individuals are within your own family. You can serve others and yourself too. Mothers can fall into the trap of self-sacrificing to the expense of their own well being and I was no exception. Sooner would have been better than later to know this for my family.

One of the ways to stop putting yourself last is to calendar an appointment with yourself to write your talents. Treat yourself the way you would want to be treated. Many a time I heard the golden rule and if you will apply this to yourself your capacity to serve those around you will be greater.

Consider this meeting with you to be as important as if you were meeting with a CEO of a successful company. If this is hard at first think of what you admire in others and it is often the case that these attributes are inside of you too. Honor this time to find the genius dwelling inside of you.

Think of similarities and differences of humans being like a chocolate chip cookie. When you go to a potluck party there could be several different kinds. Each cookie is the same kind yet different. There are 100's of wonderful recipes. Let this analogy of ingredients apply to you. Each person has their own unique combination of gifts that lead to successes that contribute to the world.

Your individual identity is of utmost importance to protect. When you start with you, it gives others permission to start to change around you. Claim who you really are and be whole!

What are a couple of big WHY's that stop the assistance before it starts?

Two main barriers that prevent many people from getting help are money and the second WHY is accessibility to good care. When it comes to mental illness many are in positions where earning income is extremely difficult, and in some cases not possible. If you are the one with the diagnosis know that what employment you can do on your own will be rewarding and worth the hurdles you will jump to get a job.

WORK IS A GIFT!

Are you searching for what kind of help is available to give you relief? The reality is that many of you will not have the resources or the people for support. Areas of a person's life such as physical, mental, emotional, intellectual and spiritual are like a puzzle that is connected.

Care for many is not affordable. Financial realities will come up and realizing your life is of great value will help with the pressures of bills. Sadly, good professional help can be costly and difficult to get. New patients are looking at a several months on a waiting list to see a good doctor. A stay in the hospital psychiatric intensive care unit can cost tens of thousands of dollars in a few weeks. In many areas there are no beds available or you have to travel long distances because there is no facility where you live.

When I was dealing with this sickness twenty plus years ago oftentimes there was very little to no coverage. Thankfully there has been laws passed to have mental illness treated like physical problem and is much more complete and inclusive with what will be paid for. The questions that were asked long ago are not asked now. In order for me to receive the vital care necessary we were required to pay a large percentage out of our own pocket. I'm glad for a husband that was able and willing to do and make the necessary sacrifices for me to receive the best care.

Since there is a shortage of good help, relieve yourself of the thinking that the profession is there to take your money and realize there are many in need that can take your place. This is a huge challenge in this particular part of the health industry and it is projected that mental illness will be an epidemic in the years to come.

At the time when this illness first surfaced there was close to zero awareness on my part and that the care I was being given was for my own good. Remember this if you are just starting out and looking for answers. Write down what you are wanting and you will be able to see more clearly the solutions when they show up. You will have criteria of who will be the best connection so you can have an honest exchange and receive feedback. If your opportunity to have quality care has been limited or nothing at all, keep your ears and eyes open for what is available in your community. Oftentimes there has been generous donors that gift services to those in need and it is FREE for you. Money is just one of the many hardships.

Over the years, more than sixty professionals have given me one on one counseling in the different areas of mental wellness. These were doctors and holistic practitioners, spiritual leaders, business coaches and mentors who are outstanding in their fields. After a long while the different plans that were suggested began to come into harmony. For example, many successful entrepreneurs go to bed early and get up early. This was totally consistent to what God has said to do in the scriptures. The same action step would come from family, doctors, business mentors, and coaches too.

Keeping unity and simplicity was important as I chose what to combine in the different plans into what would work for me. This was a process and I'll admit at first it felt like I was a ping pong ball being sent back and forth to see what was related to what. At first it was the family doctor, then then psychiatrist with a psychologist being needed too. It was wishful thinking for one doctor to be able to take care of things. Now there is an understanding that these different fields address different questions and types of care.

One doctor helps you become familiar with the medications that are available and the risks associated with them, while the other doctor is counseling you to be able to verbalize what you are going through and deal with the emotions and thoughts as they surface. It's kind of like a piano and organ, they both have keyboards but they are two very different instruments. This is the case with doctors so knowing their expertise and you will be able to communicate what you need faster and get better solutions with less frustration. This will also save time and money.

Another tip that was useful was to pretend I was wearing medical shoes and I came to know this type of work is taxing on the practitioners too. It has been my experience to have to find a new doctor often as they close their practices.

I combined the best of the best into a plan so I was able to do the work and report back the results. Patterns developed and were watched so adjustments and alignments could be made for strength in mental health and later physical wellness. What worked for me was for the doctor to explain why the drug worked this way and what it was supposed to help. Also, the risks were explained if I chose to take it or not. In the first generations of medications you would take a medicine to counteract the side effects of the medication. It would take a couple weeks to become effective so waiting until you were in a crisis was a definite consideration. Some of the medications required a blood test regularly to see the affect it was having on body organs. Sometimes the insurance will not pay and the smallest dose could cost hundreds of dollars a month.

Check with a pharmacist and they may know of how you can get financial assistance if the drug is not affordable. In the beginning it was an easier decision to take the medicine so I could be stable and be with my family. Staying in reality and focusing on what was happening in the here and now was the "what" that needed to happen at first. Dealing with long term side effects of the medicine could be dealt with later when things settled down and I was back home with my family.

What I learned is how important it is for your doctor to be able to see you when you are acting and thinking your normal self, so you can have a reasonable basis for care. This is a different approach than treating symptoms. It is being PROACTIVE rather than REACTIVE. Having this center base of facts will require a PREVENTION approach to wellness. This track record is what provided the opportunity for me to try look at options over the years and make adjustments and alignments along the way. This is one of the reasons to be wise in choosing your doctors and stay with them over a period of time. It will become easier to handle the issues and the decisions of what to do next will be clearer.

Sometimes the insurance coverage would change and it would become necessary for me to decide to pay out of pocket in order for me to stay with the same doctor who was familiar with my history. This is really important if you seek optimal health and increased options under medical supervision.

The type of doctor I was seeking would be one who would explain what the medications and treatment were for and the plus or minus of what could happen according to what I was being asked to do. This will require you to be open and honest to communicate what is going on and you'll need to have some self-awareness. Abilities to articulate this will vary and sometimes the caregivers will be trusting you and the table will turn and you will get to trust them.

My doctors keep up on the new research and medications which will open the door for new options. Percentages were discussed a lot. I was allowed to choose what range I wanted to try. For example: this med works 75% of the time, and 25% it doesn't. These statistics would be weighed out and discussed with those that were in my circle of trust. I stayed accountable for the results either way.

Taking another pair of listening ears was a good idea. Write down what you are going to do and when you will report back how you are doing. If you need help remembering what your action steps are set time aside at the appointment and have the doctor help you with a wrap up summary. Have a chart and check it off daily. Keep in mind my abilities to communicate on this level took years and I did a lot of studying on my own to understand the condition.

It is important to be realistic as you work towards the ideal.

In the field of mental health there are what is known and so many unknowns. There will be bumpy and smooth times so hold onto your hat and stay on the ride. Realize what is being asked of you is not a 100% perfect science and if you expect it to be so this will only make it harder.

Blaming and being mad at whoever will only slow your healing down and stifle your growth. One thing that was helpful was to keep the variables to a minimum by not doing too much new all at once. If you have a couple things you are trying side by side it's much easier to tell what is working.

If your intuition or awareness is off it will be better for you to trust those who are your support system and do what they recommend. **Remember this is still a choice.** If you become a danger to yourself or another you will be choosing to put yourself in a place where others will be acting for you and this is not fun. Sometimes the depth of the mental illness is such that the caregiver is placed in this difficult position right from the get go. That is when you are grateful for those who are compassionate and do their best with love. Let those you have chosen do their job and trust them!

Again, when you are wanting to choose treatments-

PREVENTION IS THE KEY PRINCIPLE.

Also, you may be asked to simplify and apply some behavior modification. This could be cutting back on what your children are involved in a letting them develop their imaginations and do activities together that will bring them closer in the end. This change of routine was a big challenge at first. Evidently from the contributions that have been written for this book from family it was a big adjustment for them too.

Are you saying "YES" to people and projects when really it would be better if you were saying "NO". After hospitalizations it became critical that I be diligent in self-care in order to serve my family first and then others. One thing that made it easier was I gained clarity on what I needed and wanted and the right opportunities and people started coming into my life. I also improved over time in being able to see and make decisions much better and faster. Set a time limit. This will put the mind at rest and keep you less distracted. Your energy will increase. Decide to Decide!

Professionals who are outside of family have the ability to separate the emotions that can come into play. When searching for help make sure you have done your due diligence to check for credibility by those who have previously worked with them as patients or clients. It's important to get good help.

Keep up as much of your normal routine as possible and at the very least include a few minutes of fun. It can be very trying for the others in the household to watch all the attention go to the one who is sick. Realize each person within the family has needs and wants. Doing nice activities with each other will be prevention for someone feeling slighted not to act out. We know there is complexity to this health condition and each case is so individual.

Explore and Experiment with the possibilities.

Action Steps

*Vocalize in advance how others can support you.

*Be proactive not reactive. What can you do to stay in prevention mode?

*Use the communication formula of red, yellow, or green to determine what kind of care is needed.

*Write questions ahead of time to ask a mentor/coach/doctor/friend.

*Make an action list with one to three things you will do and check it off daily.

*Calendar an appointment with yourself to write your talents and what you are good at. Ask others what your gifts are.

*Listen and come to an understanding.

*Ask the question am I taking things personal? If so what can you do to stop.

*Say "Yes" or "No" quickly.

*Decide to decide.

CHAPTER 2

THE GIFT OF INVESTING IN YOURSELF

THE GIFT OF INVESTING IN YOURSELF

Your wellness is priceless! Receiving health care can be financially costly and it is important to invest the time and money to be healthy. If you allow your mental condition to become life threatening here are a few examples of what can happen. Your independence could be taken as you are tied down, you'll be separated from your belongings, family, and friends, a daily uniform of a hospital gown will be your clothing, choices made for you, plus more. Visitors will go through a search from security and their valuables placed in lockers as they wait for the chance to see you for a short time each day. You will be doing everyone around you a favor if you prevent these possibilities by staying disciplined with a routine and take care of yourself.

One area that will be addressed is medication. Getting to stabilization is extremely important. Listen to your medical advisers and those close to you. Until you are grounded trust them for a season. If possible, make this part of the plan that you make ahead of time on how you will communicate that you are ready to make your own decisions. This can be really touchy so be prepared to hear what can be changed and what to accept.

YOU WILL NEED HELP FROM OTHERS

For those who want to be medication free that could be a possibility if you are willing to be medically monitored, highly disciplined with the structure of a steady morning and evening routine, exercise, and live a healthy sustainable lifestyle. With patience and discipline, you can come to a point where little or no medicine MIGHT be an option. In a way it would have been easier for me to just swallow the daily pill. Over time I've been able to do this with a lot of help from doctors who practice traditional medicine, mentors, nutritionists and holistic practitioners, family and friends.

Know the risks of being on or off medication. Go over this with your doctor AHEAD of time. Make this part of your written plan. Consider taking someone from your circle of trust to these appointments to help you remember and process the information, so you can make the best decision possible.

Mental illness has many faces and is not a respecter of persons! Whether you have money in your bank account or not, your skin white, black, pink or purple, it makes no difference. Anyone can have an experience with this. In fact, one in five Americans will have a mental health condition. (See nami.org) The numbers increase substantially that you will know or be able to interact and help someone who is going through this.

In the beginning medicine was necessary for me to take because of the severity of the state of mind and physical body. Returning to stability mentally and physically happened quickly. I realize there is a uniqueness to that in my scenario. When it comes to this choice there are people with mental illness who for various reasons will not take the medications. They find it too expensive, or they are allergic to it, that there are undesirable side effects, or the medicine is ineffective. There is a myriad of possibilities. Do what is necessary to be healthy and happy. You are a special person with or without medicine. **Let the miracle be about you being the best you can be!**

One doctor questioned the need of what was spent as there are many who offer a healing that are what you would call quack promises that lead to a below zero bank account. Questions like this from a physician or caregiver are appropriate since those who suffer from mental illness conditions can go on spending sprees or give money away too freely. I measured out the risks and was willing to try going into some uncharted territory and accept the consequences with what I spent and who worked with me.

Because of the way I accepted accountability my replies were firm in knowing that every penny has been worth it regardless if the results. If you choose to take this kind of attitude it can help you through the disappointments and losses. I have found it useful to stop comparing what does or doesn't work for me to what works for another.

 Facts are, there are too many unknowns and each one of us is so unique. Expecting every treatment, procedure, or training to work 100% all the time will cause a lot of grief and frustration. The cold hard facts are some things won't work and some will. Expect to buckle up for the wild ride at first. It will get smoother the more times you stay on the right road and keep trying.

BEGIN WHERE YOU ARE RIGHT NOW

Every human has common needs and you will have come to light what you are blind to as you start asking for help. Be careful on what you attribute to mental illness, when in reality you are having a normal mortal experience. Remember your thoughts want to keep you safe. Going into new territory will likely be met with resistance. If you are wondering if what you are going through is normal get some feedback with this from someone who has been trained to know the difference between the two.

Having your eyes opened to correct truths and principles can be life changing when applied with repetition, consistency, and discipline.

Good decisions that you are making will start producing evidence that corresponds to proper outcomes. Focus on progression and the good successes you are having from the fruits of your labors.

The time is now. You can have appropriate boundaries, be a companion, a parent, grandparent, and friend. It is possible to be a student, have a career, contribute to society, and have a life out in the world. Your dreams will become a reality as you continue to do the work.

ASK IF THE TIMING IS RIGHT?

There are those who wish they had more time as their life is busy. Those who are lonely wish they had less. Realize setbacks happen. Sometimes what you thought was the first step may be an example of the cart before the horse. What can you do with the cart if buying the horse is not what is possible yet? In other words, adjust as needed. There are many ideas and the important thing is to pick one or two of them to test and prove for results. In some cases, you can have people test two different plans at the same time to see which one works best.

Ponder what problem you want to solve? Learning to keep your schedule and activities simple is smart. Perhaps this book will help you prioritize your thoughts to be centered to time being just exactly right the way it is.

If you are saying… WHEN I HAVE:...more time...extra money…. when I retire…. when the children are grown…. I WILL DO THIS could be delaying the joy you can have now.

Consider how you want to get yourself back into the present and mindfully meditate. You may want to stop with "the grass is greener on the other side" type thinking and see your happiness soar to new heights.

DOING 1% IS 100% BETTER THAN NOTHING!

Remember, there are 60,000 plus thoughts you have in a given day. It's important to select a few of the most important. It can be a trap when you have so many things you want to do and you let time pass without choosing. A busy mind is a gift when the thoughts are managed with purpose and intention. The more often you evaluate your thinking, feelings, and emotions the easier it will become to have awareness.

When it comes to mental illness it is unlikely that you will find a magical instant cure. Sometimes it's a couple steps back to make more steps forward. Each day is about constantly learning, growing, and putting into action the knowledge you receive. That is what living is all about. That's progress!!! That's better than doing nothing at all.

I have had the opportunity to serve a friend who was in a psychiatric intensive care unit and have some insights and perspectives from both sides of being a patient as well as a caregiver. Having experience in both directions has helped with knowing how to handle my own diagnosis. After coming home from the hospital many of the decisions that I made had to do with not wanting to go to the hospital again and have my freedom taken away. Staying away from my little ones was pure torture. My children were dear to me and being restrained in a bed knowing they were being cared for by another left a hole in my heart as big as the universe.

Thankfully the hospital stays were but days even though it seemed like forever. The large loving family of mine would take rotations with me and it was only a few weeks when the children were away.

This changing season of life reminds me of sea creatures, shellfish, and the starfish that are fascinating as you learn how to live on the rough rocks. The tide ebbs in and out and the pools of water that collect at the bottom is where they live. That means they are in the hot sun during the day and the cold water at night as the fresh water crashes in throughout the twenty-four hours.

Opposition is natural and can be paralleled to sea life and in daily living. When we can wisely begin adapting and adjusting quickly to varied circumstances you build strength in character.

Find the golden lining inside of you as you pursue ways to live with faith and optimism in the storms of life!

Commonly feelings of betrayal and resentment surface from your loved one. Do you best to distance yourself from the fiery darts that may be aimed at you. Know that this is the illness coming up and give them the benefit of the doubt when you can.

Humans basic desire is to be free, being tied down in a psychiatric ward goes contrary to that. An individual's freedom of choice is so fundamental that when it is taken away there are feelings that come up. Keep in mind these may start to surface when the hospitalization is over.

You may notice they resent or wonder why you did what you did. The medical treatments are hard. Maybe one day they'll get the reasons for why the situation was handled the way it was and maybe not. If you are a caregiver take comfort when you know you did the best you could in a hard situation you didn't ask for.

The greatest gift you can give is your time and listen to understand as long as you're able to. One thing that is vital, is to allow the person to do as much as they can for themselves and get on their own two feet.

Action Steps

Ask yourself these questions and save time:

*What you can eliminate?

*Fix?

*Change?

*Do without?

*Track your thoughts and feelings. Do you notice patterns?

*Who can you take to appointments that can help you make important decisions?

*What good fruits are coming into your life from your labors?

CHAPTER 3

THE GIFT OF ONENESS IN YOUR SOUL

THE GIFT OF ONENESS IN YOUR SOUL

Oneness in your soul is about having the most important relationship within yourself. The meaning of ONENESS in the Merriam-Webster dictionary is-: the state of being completely united with or a part of someone or something, a person's total self. Tranquility in the soul is having the mind and body learning to master the fleshy physical side of our existence along with the spiritual and mental coming into harmony. Can you honestly say you are full of peace, joy, and happiness?

An important question is-

ARE YOU TAKING AS GOOD OF CARE OF YOURSELF AS YOU DO FOR OTHERS?

In the King James Bible the scripture says- "And he answering said, Thou shalt love the Lord thy God with all thy heart, and with all thy soul, and with all thy strength, and with all thy mind; and thy neighbor as thyself." (Luke 10:27)
Let's consider the two words AS THYSELF.

How are you doing with that? Do you love yourself as the divine person that you are? When you are serving others are you running around like a chicken with its head cut off?

Busy...Busy... Busy... Can you really effectively help another when you are going about life in a crazy way? The answer to the last question could be that as you continue with this fast pace problems with relationships, health, or money, may start showing up where you will have to STOP OR BE STOPPED.

When your soul is in a state of oneness you will find you are being charitable and able to take care of your needs as well. Be whole with yourself in mind, body, heart, and soul.

SELF CARE IS NOT SELFISH

To put the principle of self-care into context here is a story of a young man sharing about how much he loved his mother. She would be up early until late, serving to physical and mental exhaustion. She would let time get away from her by not preparing and eating healthy meals. The love for her family was unending and genuine until one day her heart stopped beating. Life seemed to take an unfair twist, as now her son was attending her funeral as a young boy. Oh, how he wished she would have lived a long healthy life and got to know her grandchildren. It was heartbreaking to hear him express how his mother would take care of everyone one else at the expense of her own health and family and was the most selfish thing she could have done. He missed her terribly.

Learning how to care for our precious bodies is so important. Mothers are caring nurturers and often fall into a trap of forgetting to remember to take care of their basic health requirements. One of those basic needs is allowing ourselves some rest and down time.

Another good question to ask yourself is- What is your sleep patterns?

If insomnia is plaguing you enough to seek good medical attention this sleep will likely come up. Especially when it comes to how you are managing stress even when you are physically sick. Stress and sleep can often be connected. Pay attention to see when you are asked about this right at the beginning. It's been my experience that those who are seasoned in what they do will make this question a priority. Mental well-being and thoughts will be much clearer when you are on schedule with your sleep.

A lot of times you hear about rising early in the AM to improve your life. What if your emphasis was on the PM? It makes sense if you retire before it is late that it will be much easier to rise. If you are tempted to think you can stay up late because you can sleep late and still get the same results of vim and vigor, think of a farmer and his cows. The farmer and the cows know they are milked consistently every day first thing in the morning to receive the milk. Some people may need to adjust if working at night but regardless there is a certain amount of time the body will need to regenerate and getting into a rhythm is important.

Little babies and elderly can get their days and nights mixed up and this can happen with those who have mental illness. After a thorough physical is given and no body malfunction is specifically identified, then start to address sleep.

Research is showing 7-9 hours is a healthy amount. Are you in that range? If your patterns are really off take a 24- hour period and start to write when you wake up and go to sleep. Take 15-minute increments and increase or decrease the time you lay down and adjust accordingly. This way you can get back to a proper pattern if you are sleeping too much or too little. When you are back on schedule provide yourself the structure in the morning and evening to stay steady and disciplined. Soon you should have a solid block of sleep. Focus on your PM routine FIRST and your early AM routine will fall into place much easier. Having a consistent PM (night routine) is crucial and will make a major difference in having peaceful thoughts and feelings. Who is all about reducing unhealthy stress in your life?

Action Steps

*Start tracking SLEEP FIRST by writing down when you go to bed and rise. (add what you eat and drink later)

*Set your alarm the night before and have integrity with yourself by getting up.

*Establish a nightly PM routine to quiet the mind.
*What is your morning AM routine?

 UNDERSTAND THE POWER OF YOUR SOUL

Think of yourself as special and sacred. When you go on vacation and visit cathedrals or temples they are treated with care and reverence. They are kept clean. Do you treat your body the same?

One of the big signals to those that love you is when they notice you are going days without showering or changing your clothes. Your hair becomes greasy and you stink. Take charge of your body and how you treat it. Notice your hair and nails and care for them in order to send out a message that you are ready to do the simple daily disciplines.

Choose a certain time when you will be dressed and ready to go out and meet people at the start of the day. If you have a box to check of daily you will have the ability to notice progress. If you notice several boxes left unmarked this can notify you that depression is starting so you can stop the cycle more quickly. Other areas of your life will start coming into order so inspiration and creativity will start flowing once again in a positive direction.

*Keep yourself clean. (Bathe regularly, do your hair and nails, etc.)

*Create words that you hear daily that are positive. Examples are-
My body is being strengthened in every way now.
Every little cell in my body is happy and healthy.

WHAT IS YOUR BODY PARTAKING OF?

You may find out you have nutritional deficiencies or allergies. Watching your drinking and eating patterns is very important. This will give many clues as to the reason you are thinking and feeling the way you are.

EATING AND DRINKING CRAP = FEELING LIKE CRAP

Are you rushing around and cramming food into your mouth without paying attention? Look for patterns of when you choose to eat unhealthy or healthy. This could be in times of stress when you emotionally eat or even in times when you are celebrating when you start gobbling down sweet temptations. If you know you are going to a party, plan ahead by taking your own food or go with a full stomach.

The opposite can also manifest into a problem with meal skipping. If you find yourself in too big a hurry to have regular meals have the food in the fridge ready. You can place a picture on the mirror to strategically remind you to go get a bite of what you have made. Set an alarm if necessary. This keeps you on regular schedule.

I have a picture of our family eating at my parent's home where our spirits were fed emotionally and mentally as we sat in the kitchen eating delicious fruits and vegetables as we visited. Convenience and availability is the key to what you will put in your tummy. Plan ahead!

At a mindfulness meditation class one of the exercises was to bring your lunch and spend 3 hours eating it. At first it was "are you kidding me"? This was definitely a first. Learning to enjoy food by noticing the texture, the sound, the taste, the feeling, and minimize the distractions was really insightful in ways to improve.

There are many cultures where the family is gathered around sitting at the kitchen table listening to each other. Setting time aside to eat will strengthen relationships.

Because eating became a big problem that affected my mental and physical stability in the past the importance of having healthy regular meals is part of my wellness routine now. This attitude evolved after hearing how the doctors tried to treat my symptoms with IV's etc. The hospitalization became necessary because of the rapid decline of my body and mind in a very short amount of time. I was literally dying from the inside out.

My family was concerned and there was mighty prayer and fasting in my behalf. My problem was thinking I was in a position to do the same. This is what started the downward spiral from the lack of eating. I had zero awareness of the problem. The seriousness of the situation was not realized until after I came home and was stable and began asking the family what had happened.

Life threatening issues started to come up. The food and liquid wouldn't digest and stay down. My state of mind was so busy and thoughts going so fast that days could go by without eating properly. First and foremost was the urgency to get me drinking consistently, then came the eating. There came a point where it was necessary for my meals to be prepared by others.

Love in the home environment was where I thrived and healed. As my condition improved I was able to make food side by side with a family member until gradually I was able to cook on my own.

One of the keys to success is to know ahead. Meeting with a nutritionist and going to classes is a good idea. **Education on how to improve became a lifeline.**

Reflecting on what I was able to do before the health problems started became the new goals of where to get back to. What kept me going was the desire to nourish my own family with home cooked meals, nature walks, hosting small family gatherings and enjoying the simple joys of life. Stretch yourself to be as independent as possible.

Remember you are capable and trust yourself!

One thing to know is you can rise above what is going on whether you have a supportive family or not. There are many wonderful people in the history books that have been through brutal injustices, less than the ideal circumstances, and still rose above all the heartache. Why there is such unfairness and inequality in the world can be hard to understand. Let it be known my heart goes out to you if this is the case. Just know there can be inner peace and oneness in your soul regardless of the circumstance you find yourself in.

Even when doing good works and living life with good intention you are still human and susceptible to adversity. Think of the many leaders who went through so much. Christ was perfect and what did he do to be spit upon, beaten and crucified? Gandhi, a peacemaker, was assassinated. Mother Teresa who lived with many ailments throughout her life, continued to serve the poor. The first black president of Africa, Nelson Mandela, was imprisoned for twenty-seven years even after he had given much of his wealth to better the lives of children. If your life has been one of pain and long suffering, that visits frequently as an unwelcome guest, you can carry on. Know that "the bitter cup will pass" for sweeter days ahead!

Another remedy during tough times is laughter that truly is medicine for the soul. Stick around those who help you lighten up and find humor in even serious matters.

Action Steps

*Write WHO you trust and come to an agreement of what will happen if you need medical attention.

*Find someone who will watch for the signs when you are neglecting your body and will help you.

*Ask the person you want there for support if they have _____ minutes of time to help you. If not now, then when.

*Write down the problem and set a time when you will have a solution. (If no answer is clear after doing the work to make a final decision go over when you will put the situation on the shelf and have more information.)

* Calendar time to prepare and eat meals. Provide the time for yourself as if you are an important client.

*Early in the week decide a menu for at least five breakfasts, lunches, and dinner meals.

Tips for caregivers

*Consider taking a nutritional class together.

*Plan a time when you can go food shopping and prepare meals side by side.

PLAN YOUR PLAY/EXERCISE

Nature is a great way to get some sun, fresh air, and to SEE what's around you. Physical exercise stimulates the good feelings and emotions to process the experiences we are going through in healthy and appropriate ways.

This story of one of my mentors who has many successful businesses and teaches people how to celebrate and have playful fun. I was on my way to the appointment and daily life was full of the unexpected. Time was filled with taking care of the needs of loved ones who we were grateful to have staying with us, as a dear relative had a sudden accident and died. Shock was the feeling we were left with as we adjusted to the fact that she was physically not with us anymore. It was comforting to know there was no suffering and she was in a heavenly place.

When I arrived, my mentor was quick to take note of body language and had a wise intuition of exactly what was needed. A few tender tears were allowed to fall as I took some time to process the loss which I hadn't allowed myself the time to do. It was very healing to know I had someone by my side that was there to encourage and was without judgment. This was a special time to care for and replenish strength so I could continue to serve others. The appointment turned into a field trip at the park. I was told to give myself permission to play and have fun! The swings were right there and I was able to feel the fresh air on a beautiful day.

She was swinging right beside me and the laughter was great. We took off our dress shoes and put the grass under our feet. It felt good to be grounded to Mother Earth and the beauty that was all around. What others thought, and the cares of the world, were put aside for the next couple of hours. Take note the mentor was BESIDE and WITH me along the way. Finding someone to be humorous WITH you instead of AT you, are a true friend.

Wow, it was a bit of a challenge and stretch at first. At first, I will admit I was silent and thinking about the money I paid for the appointment and was a bit skeptical. Doing a field trip to the park for business was the last thing I ever would have guessed to work. Investing time and money to celebrate was worth it! I felt better right away, but it was the following day where I really noticed a huge difference in how I was thinking and feeling.

Learning you get your work done and processing emotions too as you are playing was insightful. Working with a positive attitude made the chores get done faster and easier. The mental clarity was incredible! Then and there, I decided to do this again and change the normal scheduling of appointments to be mixed calendaring, planned fun, and celebrations.

Refreshing by un-scheduling your "need to do list", into scheduling your "want to do list" first, helped with the speed of what was getting done. **Play Makes the World-Go-Round and the work fun.**

Action Steps

*Are you calendaring fun things to look forward to along with your work?

*First thing in the morning decide when you are going to physically get your body moving. And for how long.

*Who can play and celebrate with you?

*Do you know a mentor that is good at both work and play? When that person comes to mind when will you connect with them?

RELEASING EMOTION WITH MUSIC

Music and vibration can make you feel happy or sad. Getting up and doing some movement is great for the body too. The dissonant notes stir a different kind of emotion that is different or hurts the ears. You think NO that's not right. This could be compared to experiences of life.

Sometimes the notes hurt. You want a different sound to be there and to your surprise it resolves out and makes sense when it is all over.

Healing can take place as you listen to emotional music and let those tears fall. The salt in tears is healing. The release is a good way to let feelings out in a healthy way to be better. We take out physical garbage every day so letting go of emotional garbage makes sense too. Life is life, and there are appropriate times to let those eyes leak. In the beginning the doctors' appointments were really rough. My stomach would be in knots and hearing the bipolar diagnosis was painful at first and managing the condition the rest of my life was the last thing I wanted to hear. Couldn't it all go away?

After this kind of depressing news from the doctor I would go home and be alone and listen to music that would bring peace to my soul. At first it would be a song to move me to tears. There is a particular song about the woman in the Bible who had the issue of blood that I would listen to. This story reminded me that yes, I have something to deal with, and to keep having faith. One day all people will be healed through God and everything will be perfect and beautiful once again.

Emotional release is important to do in appropriate ways. Through the generations of one side of my family, tears were stopped before they could start because they didn't want to be seen crying. This was the case at funerals too. Later I came to be educated to know that showing emotion is healthy. Sometimes society perpetuates a stigma that by allowing your feeling to process you are weak. It can be hard to know what to say when someone is sad, so try seeing if stillness and moments of silence calms your loved one.

I'd take a look in the mirror, smile, and after splashing some cold water on my face was renewed and refreshed after 5 min. After the melancholy songs the emotions would be balanced with a few uplifting ones such as "Let the Sun Shine In". Take note of your moods and watch for a shift.

Know that if one person can make lemonade out of lemons, so can you! Music is great for the body and keeping your chin up and keeping a smile. Quiet time and soft music is soothing to the soul.

Watching the children dance and use their talents was really funny and super exercise. I found the children literally sang me back to life. Vibration and movement can be freeing as you dance. Energy will flow and you can start to feel better. Read the words to the songs first so you can choose carefully and intentionally create the atmosphere and emotion inside you. Using the whole brain is a very powerful cause for change. After the musical pick me up, get ready to carry on for the day.

Find a way to incorporate music into your life.

Action Steps

*Do you have different types of songs for your play list? (sad, happy, exercise, etc.)

*When will you have a good cry?

*Learn to play an instrument.

*Decide what emotion you intentionally want to create with music.

*Read the lyrics to the songs before you listen.

Tips for caregivers

*Ask if they would like to share playlists.

*Find a time to dance or exercise to music together.

CHAPTER 4

THE GIFT OF PLANNING SUCCESS

THE GIFT OF PLANNING SUCCESS

When something comes up out of the blue and throws a curve ball do your best to stay in the game. Make a plan. When you do this, it will help you stay avoid confusion, being overwhelmed, or paralysis by analysis, plus more. The results from searching for improvement and knowledge, has been worth the time, the ups and downs, and pain to live life fully.

Adjustments and Alignments are easier to deal with when a map of where you are headed is in place. This will help you remember what you agreed and committed to do.

A great famous quote:

"By failing to prepare, you are preparing to fail." Benjamin Franklin

When you find the person that has everything turn out perfectly the way they thought it would, 100% of the time, be sure to let them know to enter the book of all-time records or the museum for the world famous.

Here are a couple more beautiful quotes that illustrate how failures can be successes too.

Helen Keller and Benjamin Franklin lead the way when it came to overcoming obstacles.

"Making a mistake is falling down, failure is not getting back up again."

Helen Keller

"Do not fear mistakes. You will know failure. Continue to reach out."

 Benjamin Franklin

Think of going to the gym and you know the muscles you want to target and strengthen. You want to increase your stamina. Understanding where you are at and where you want to go will help your trainer know what kind of workouts and plan to give you so you see results. Visualize your experience.

BEGIN KNOWING YOUR FINISH LINE

If you are one of those people who takes a long time to make a decision, you will want to remember indecision is a decision too. The more time you stay in limbo land without saying "yes" or "no" the more energy you will be required to have. An answer of "Maybe", "I'll let you know", "I'm not sure" are tough places to be for long periods of time. There are appropriate times to know when to hold and wait. However, do yourself and others a favor and make a decision one way or the other whenever possible.

Are you able to articulate what you want? So often we can list off what we don't want without being clear on what we do want. Being able to express what your desires in areas of health, communication, relationships, career, financial, and so on will be helpful when you're deciding what to do.

Choose to focus on one idea at a time and start with your strong areas first. When you get stronger and stronger, then it will be easier to go after the weakest area to achieve sustainable success. When you speak up you may be surprised to find others who are dealing with the same kind of feelings, even though the specifics of the circumstance are different.

In order to know what to discuss, seek to vocalize the possible solutions that can be put to action now. Then you will know if what you are talking about is worth the time and energy.

When you are hurting or blue it is so easy to allow your focus to wander onto the business of others. If you enjoy serving others do you understand what they want and do you have their permission? Do you wait long enough for them to ask for help and allow them the opportunity to find solutions on their own?

There is a saying "Mind your own business" that teaches this principle. Weather it's another person, family, career, or community knowing what YOUR business is will help you recognize the right opportunities you want to be involved in and when to say yes and when to say no and who to help.

There is a story about the difference between a billionaire and a millionaire. The millionaire would say yes to almost everything and the billionaire knew exactly what he was looking for and would say "No" most of the time recognizing the exact moment to say "YES". Learning when to answer what way will pay dividends. Delegating will lighten your load too.

This is a quote of mine that comes in handy. "I am not the only leaf on the tree", meaning: if the timing is off, others are capable. It's amazing how things have a way of working out when you are open to letting people come into your circle of influence that are there for you through thick and thin.

In God's perfect timing the circle of connections will start to link up one at a time and come together. The payoff will come for those willing to do the work with patience. There are ways you can record the intangible results of inner peace and love too. The world wants to SEE outward results when the UNSEEN is of great value too. There is great benefit when both are recognized.

Action steps

*Write-I want more of …and the first step is …

*Divide your lists into intangible and tangible then prioritize into long and short-term goals.

*Set a date when you will make a decision to put the plan into action.

*Brainstorm the resources that are needed for the FIRST step that you know you will take.

*Start with a success that is doable in thirty days and break it down in four sections to complete in one month. (If this is too much at first you can start by completing a weekly goal.)

*Decide when you will come back and check on what is working, what can be better, and what you want to eliminate.

*Each week record your successes in a book where you have access to read them nightly. This gives your mind something positive to go over in your slumbers.

Tips for the caregiver

*Calendar time and listen to what they are learning.

*Provide a simple way they can report when they have completed what they have committed to do.

Contribution Family-Daughter

The person who has the greatest impact on my life is my Mom. A few years ago, my Mom was diagnosed with a disease called Bipolar. This is a brain disorder that causes unusual shifts in a person's mood, energy, and ability to function. It has been hard for our whole family to deal with, but it's helped us become closer. Through interacting with my Mom you'd never be able to tell she has Bipolar. She is always thinking about others before she thinks about herself.

Happiness beams off her face no matter how she is feeling. With the determination she has within, this disease will not slow her down. She has raised seven children and she is an amazing person. Through her example she has impacted my life and inspired me to be a better person.

CHAPTER 5

THE GIFT OF CHANGE AND GROW

THE GIFT OF CHANGE AND CHARACTER DEVELOPMENT

LEARN TO PREVENT, PREPARE, MAINTAIN, AND SUSTAIN.

Your future is bright! Plan and prepare to become even better. Being able to find light IN the darkness becomes a way to develop integrity of character. When you cry out to God instead of asking for your troubles to go away, ask for the strength to have the qualities to endure well. Ask for guidance and direction to know the principles and attributes that come along with the answers you are seeking.

The best counsel you will receive will be simple truths. **Be careful not to throw the idea out the window since it "sounds easy".**

SELF-MASTERY REQUIRES TIME

An example would be if you had a fitness coach who asks you to write in a journal every day, the hour you go to bed. There may be a time you are out late and think you'll do it later. You may find it difficult to tell your coach and have to hear the repercussions. Do it anyway.

Your change and growth will occur much faster when you follow through. When you think you will take care of it, you'll learn to have your actions match your words. In order to have a sustainable lifestyle that is rich with joy will require discipline, consistency, and commitment.

Do what you say you will

Be Yourself and say-

I BELIEVE,

I TRUST,

AND I LOVE MYSELF.

With time and patience, a negative experience will be turned to a positive one if you allow it. Stay accountable by repeating:

I Choose to…I want to…I get to…

A strength can be when you admit you are new at what you are doing and eager to seek knowledge and quickly put what you learn into action. Let go of fear and stop hesitation and decide. It's totally ok and even probable that you will make mistakes along the way. The important thing is that you are taking the shots and know that some o them will make the targets.

Acting on simple truths, recording, and sharing how you are coming along may be a hassle in the beginning, yet will save you a lot of grief in the end. Do you ready to have answers to the problem you are blind to?

Can you be open minded and teachable?

You will come to know the appropriate ways to embrace the experience and let the ebbs and tides of life flow with greater ease.

MINDFULLY MEDITATE

As you mindfully meditate you become familiar with the process of formally sitting yourself and quieting down. It becomes a way of stepping out of the busy world and STOPPING to focus on what is going around you right now.

This becomes and exercise of the mind to become comfortable by closing the eyes, and in a simple way focus on the breath. WHEN THE MIND WANDERS WHICH IT WILL, STOP, and be glad you noticed and go back to the breath and the present moment.

Meditation inspires change. It can be done regardless of what is going as you learn the skill to still the mind when troubled waters come up in life. Set time aside and put this important appointment with yourself on the calendar. You will increase and expand your abilities to manage stress instead of going into unhealthy distress.

Consider you have tens of thousands of thoughts a day so obviously you are not going to be able to act out on all of them. The brain can and will visualize the thoughts you dwell on as if they are real. Repetitive thoughts are the ones that will likely become applied into your daily life.

Here is an exercise that you can try and add your own imagination to this narrative to have your mind and body reach its highest potential. This requires only a few minutes of time a day.

Guided imagery is also a way to wind down when the time is not right to sit in a formal setting. This would be a possible example of a way to use your imagination.

Think of yourself climbing a mountain and feeling the ground under your feet and the sun penetrating through your body with comforting warmth. You go higher and higher as one foot leads the other. The breeze on your face is stimulating as the air goes in and out of your nose and expands into your lungs and out the mouth. Each peak fills you with light from the top of the head clear down through the toes. Each body part has a turn to be focused on and feels invigorated and refreshed. Notice your outside surroundings as the wind rustles the leaves in the trees and you hear the music of the birds...And so on....

Teach your thoughts to become still and listen. When you put space in between words or use two words with different spellings and meanings you will discover this effective in giving your subconscious an opportunity to give the body guidance and improvement. For example- "My mind is obedient and minds". ENLIGHTEN to IN LIGHT IN. (You are letting light in and this can be to ground you on the inside or comfort you, light in to find humor, etc.) (GOLDEN-YOU ARE GOLD IN. You are worth more than gold.)

BE A MASTER BUILDER OF YOUR DESTINY

Action Steps

*Calendar the time to Meditate.

*Write your own visualization that gives your body and opportunity for guidance and improvement.

*Say: I Choose to...I want to...I get to...

*Write three small things in the evening that will build character.

*Celebrate success in simple ways: (yell, yahoo, sing or a happy dance)

*What character trait and values are you wanting to develop more of?

*Reach out to those you know and ask them to share qualities about you.

*Seek out one confirmation of your own to recognize your growth.

*What ONE step are you going to apply and When?

~Contribution-Son-in-Law~

CPR for the Soul

Mentally altered state from addictions and the saving Love of Family and Above

I am a 43-year-old agent for an insurance company in Utah. I became addicted to heroin and other drugs and began stealing from my father to support this habit. I grew up in a respected Mormon family, in The Church of Jesus Christ of Latter-day Saints (LDS), and desperately wanted to live a cleaner life, but felt powerless over the drugs. Then one day, I walked up a mountain behind my father's house and experienced a transcendent, transforming, life-changing encounter with God that healed my addiction and helped me gain clarity for the first time in my life.

By the age of 23, I was an addict, such a mess. I was taking so many pills — "cousins" to heroin...

whatever I could get my hands on. My father is a successful dentist, and I put myself on his payroll, although he didn't notice. I was taking checks out of his mail and cashing them. I stole tens of thousands of dollars from him. His CPA is the one who realized the money was missing.

There is a beautiful movie called Pleasure Unwoven: An Explanation of the Brain Disease of Addiction. It's a documentary DVD produced in 2010 that explains that addicts just can't stop using, stealing and destroying themselves. I highly recommend it to anyone who has an addiction and anyone who is trying to help an addict. I used to walk to the store and steal things, crying because I couldn't stop myself. That's how bad it was. I lost my car, my job and everything else. I just wanted to die because I couldn't stop this body from walking around to commit crimes just to get high again.

I have an identical twin brother, and we have a younger brother. One day, my younger brother called me on the phone and said, "Dad found out you've been stealing money from him. He's on his way over to your house right now."

I had been in jail a few times, and I said, "I am not going to prison. I'm going to Mexico." So I packed a bag and was getting ready to leave. My dad pulled in the driveway and got out of the car. I began to cry, and I looked at him with dark, sorrowful pity. A horrid emptiness engulfed me. I felt like a damned soul. I didn't even believe in God at that time. My dad was the only latch I had to my old life because my twin brother was using drugs, too. And there he was. I didn't want to get close to him because I didn't know if he was going to try to tackle me or keep me from leaving. I just didn't want to go to prison.

I told my dad, "I cannot tell you how sorry I am. You're looking at somebody who's out of control. I am going to go to Mexico, and I will probably die." In my mind, the only way out was to kill myself. In fact, I had already attempted suicide, but my brother stopped me.

Dad's eyes started to fill with tears, and he told me, "No, no! Just calm down. We'll take care of this. We'll work it out. Don't go anywhere; don't do anything. Just come home. You're going to come home. I'm going to get you out of this deep hell you're in, but you're going to live by my rules. And you're going to go to church with me."

What an amazing human he is. I had already failed at rehab several times and stolen maybe $35,000 from him, yet he took me back in, like the Prodigal Son.

I moved back home, and he wanted me to wake up each morning and read Scriptures with him, go to church with him on Sunday and sit in on the family prayers. I wanted to turn my life around, but I just couldn't stop popping the pills. I started lying to my dad again.

One Tuesday evening, I got back to my dad's house after work, and I wanted to go to a bar or a club. I borrowed his truck and drove to a nearby city to pick up a friend of mine, J.P.. He was a pothead. He loved smoking pot and studying Buddhism. He was into different things every week. J.P. loved going against society and the grain. He told me two missionaries were going to be at his house in a little while to talk to him.

I said, "Let's just go!"

He said, "No, if you want me to go to the club with you, you're going to sit here and wait until these guys are done. I've got an appointment with them."

I protested. "Just leave them. These kids are twenty years old. Why are you going to meet with them? Do you just want to mess with them and tell them Santa Claus isn't real? They're not hurting anybody, and they're not addicted to stuff, so leave them alone. You just want to smoke your pot, trip out on them, Bible-bash them and try to take away their faith."

J.P. said, "No, I don't. Just shut up. Get out of here if you don't want to wait for me."

He was the only person who would hang out with me, so I waited. The two missionaries showed up. This kid from Delaware sat down and started talking to J.P.. Then he turned to me and started lighting up — I can't even explain it. He started telling me about Jesus Christ. I had heard it all before because my dad was religious.

"What Kind of Drug Is This?"

But this was incredible. It was powerful. The Spirit was speaking to me. The young missionary told me, "You are going to change. You're going to influence thousands of people. You're going to do great things — I can see it."

He prophesied my life. The room seemed to glow. I wondered if I was tripping on LSD or something because it was so potent. I wondered, "What kind of drug is this? This light and this hope…" It's like I had been in a dark cave, and somebody ripped the top off the cave, and all this light came pouring down on me. It was a beautiful feeling that went clear through me. I knew what he was saying was true.

The Spirit was burning through the room so strongly. The missionary said, "Can you feel that? That's the Spirit!" Caught up in the overwhelming transformation taking place, he stood up and shouted, "I have never felt it this strong! Wahooooo!"

Something in me changed at that moment. I was still addicted to drugs, but my heart started beating again. The missionary told me, "I want you to go to church, even if you're sedated."

I told him, "I can't do that. It's rude to go to church while I'm high."

He disagreed strongly. So I made a commitment that I would keep going to church with my dad on Sundays. There were times when I'd walk into church, even though I had just popped a bunch of pills. I was like, "I'm here. I'm barely here, but I'm here. I'm sorry I'm wasted. I'm sorry I'm high, but I'm here, and I'm going to continue on this pattern. I am going to turn my life around."

My Mountaintop Salvation Experience:

For the next six months, I tried to quit my addiction and be the man I knew I should be. One day, I got off the bus from work and saw an unfamiliar car in front of my dad's house. I thought it was a parole officer. I wondered if maybe I had forgotten to pay a ticket.

I didn't want to find out. It was 5 o'clock in the afternoon, and I decided to go for a walk, up the mountain behind my dad's house. I saw one of our neighbors, and he asked how I was doing. He said, "I see you at church. Listen, I don't know exactly what you're going through, but all I know is that you've got to give it to the Savior."

I asked, "What do you mean?"

He said, "You've just got to ask Him to take it from you."

We talked for about 15 minutes. Then I walked down the road about a mile. There were no houses out there. My dog, Scruffy, was with me. She saw the whole thing. I looked out across the valley. It was pure daylight, and I got on my knees. I had a conversation with God. I said, "I feel like there's something on the other side. I feel these little pieces of gold that have come into my life over the past six months, like what the missionary said to me. But I can't shake this addiction. I know I'm going to go use pills tonight. I know I'm going to go do whatever I can to just get loaded again. I know You can hear me. I can't do it. You've got to take it from me because I can't do it on my own."

I really didn't want to live anymore. I didn't want to disappoint my dad, who was trying to save my life. I figured I was hooked for life and would die an addict.

At that moment, I felt like someone placed hands on my head. I felt the presence of two people, whom I knew. It felt so familiar. As soon as they touched my head, I knew everything was going to be OK. They felt like brothers. I sensed that they had always been there, had always been in charge and were doing the work of God. Everything was clear. I knew Jesus Christ was the Savior. But the sensation I had wasn't of realizing something; it was a sensation of remembering something, and how could I have forgotten that?

I didn't actually see people standing there with me, but I sensed their overwhelming presence. It was the Spirit testifying. You can't testify about truth and not feel its power. I realized a lot of things that day. When it all peeled back, I remembered that God is so involved in our lives as we're doing our everyday things, and we can't see it. But for a moment, I saw it.

For some reason, I had a pen and paper with me, and I wrote down 20 truths, or lessons, God gave me to strengthen me and overcome my addiction. They were things like, "Don't dwell on anything but the truth of God." The truth of God means that you should work hard to support your family. Another truth is that we should talk good about our neighbors instead of talking bad about them. Just doing good unto others. Everything that's worthwhile, that's where you dwell. That's what you put your mind on.

During this mountaintop experience, I saw my addiction clearly — and it cured me. Addicts know what's going on, but they're so scatterbrained. This experience rebuilt my mind. I stopped taking drugs at that moment, and I never even had withdrawals — no shaking, no nothing. I looked out across the valley, and I saw the intricate involvement of heaven pouring through everything.

I felt an inextinguishable love and felt how deeply we are all connected. We are certainly never alone.

A New Beginning

After this phenomenal experience, I walked down the mountain, back into my dad's house. He was there, and I asked him who had visited. He said it was a friend of his. It wasn't a cop, like I had feared. He looked at me. He could tell there was something different about me.

I said, "Dad, I'm going to be honest with you. I have continued to do drugs while I've lived here, but it's gone now. I'm telling you, it's all gone!"

I walked toward him and hugged him. I felt so carefree and happy again, like I did when I was 12 years old. Finally, my brain was in the right place. Everything had hope in it again. Life was beautiful. I went to my room and typed out the 20 truths that God had shared with me on the mountaintop — truths that He had custom-tailored just for me. Twenty years later, I still have that list of the 20 keys to my sobriety.

But even though my brain was fixed, I knew I needed to repay the money I owed my dad and begin serving myself and others as I would serve God Himself. I knew I had to take control of my life, or the devil would do so again.

I decided to go on a two-year mission trip to Atlanta for the Mormon church, the LDS church. I wanted to give back. I wasn't married yet, and I didn't have kids yet. The leaders in the church weren't sure they wanted me to be a missionary. They didn't want me relapsing out there, away from home, and setting a bad example for others.

But then one of the top leaders read my file and told me he wanted me to go. He said, "You've been through a lot."

I said, "Yeah."

And he said, "No, you've really been through a lot!" His eyes seemed to look right to the core of my soul. After only a moment, he proclaimed, "You are going to make a great missionary!" The Lord helped him see, without words, the purification of Christ's atonement.

CPR for the Soul

One day, I was talking to my friend, Greg, a phenomenal guy. I stopped him and said, "Hey, Greg. You have some friends who have gone back to using, but you've always stayed good. Your friends kind of fell back into the pit. They're like the pig that eats its own vomit. How can I avoid doing that?"

Greg told me, "You've got to do three things: you've got to show up once a week and meet with other people, talk about God — you've got to go to church. Second, you've got to pray every day. Show some respect — get down on your knees. You can't be lying in bed. It takes maybe ten seconds or thirty seconds. And third, you've got to read just one verse of Scripture every day. It has to be a meaningful one, and a different one every day. You'll never fall too far if you just do those three things and never miss. The Lord loves consistency!"

Then I realized that those three important activities form the acronym CPR: church (every Sunday), prayer (every day, on your knees) and reading Scriptures (at least one per day). I worked three jobs to go on the mission trip in Atlanta. I went out there and shared with people what I know: CPR for the soul — it's the consistency that counts!

Life Is Grace, and Pain Is a Gift

Life is grace. God has put us on this Earth so we can learn. Every bit of pain we go through helps us understand the object and design of our existence, which is happiness. It is only by His grace that we get to be here.

The pain we feel in our lives is a gift. You cannot comprehend the beauty of daylight and sunshine until you've been in Alaska in the wintertime for three months straight, and you come back down to California and see the green grass and feel the warm sunshine.

To anybody in pain, I want to tell you that we are all in the middle of a process. How do we find truth? It's not that hard, but it is a process. We have to build our spiritual "muscle." If you want to do some pull-ups, you don't just start doing a bunch of them right away if you've never done them before. If you try to skip that growth process and ask God to give you strength without going through the pain, then you have missed the whole point of life. Why would the Lord rob us of the process?

Here are just two of many Bible verses that I turn to when I need to feel God's strength:

"But seek ye first the kingdom of God, and his righteousness; and all these things shall be added unto you."

— MATTHEW 6:33

"For every one that asketh receiveth; and he that seeketh findeth; and to him that knocketh it shall be opened."

— MATTHEW 7:8

CHAPTER 6

THE GIFT OF INTENTION AND COMMITMENT

THE GIFT OF HONEST INTENTION AND COMMITMENT

What are you focusing and dwelling on?

Let's consider a doughnut and ask yourself the question-Do you want to focus on the yummy pastry that is there or the hole? There is a time and a place for both. When you choose to focus on the doughnut or in other words what you do have you will do one simple action step daily that you've already learned and know what's next. The hole represents the mystery, what you want to learn and the new knowledge you are seeking.

If you just went through something would you like to evaluate the situation so the same story isn't repeated a little bit louder and a whole lot worse? Your exploration of the mystery may require some patience as you take the time to enjoy the journey. Once you figure out what you are blind too you know you are illuminated and that's a new kind of yummy. Once you have the knowledge you will find getting back to work fun. Those small steps add up and will make a big difference over time. Noticing all chain reaction of goodness with gratitude will lighten your load along the way and applying what you have learned and getting to work will be fun!

CONTINUE AND COMPLETE

A mentor gave me an example of a mountain that has a tunnel that was made to get you THROUGH point A to point B. You are in the light and stepping forward into the darkness with the knowledge that this will save time and is safer than going around or climbing up the mountain. You know it is bright on the opposite side and even though stepping into the darkness with faith can be a bit scary, it is worth going the distance.

Knowing that you are capable is important. Your actions will speak volumes over your words. This is a time to decide with purpose and intention of what you are willing to do or not do.

Review the conversation and commit to the one gem of wisdom that you are going to apply and be wise and follow through when you have completed what you said you would. One of the mentors would make a small list of the daily basics with a little place to put a check. This helped with consistency. This chart was made at the close of the appointment and was the wrap up. It was helpful to have something I could see and carry. Also, being asked what step was next and commit to taking it by the next day created forward momentum.

What you hear, say, see, write, and report on and evaluate will turn into success at a much higher and faster rate.

Here are a couple of examples of saying and wanting cake and eating it too. Entitlement and laziness easily creep in. This is a couple of examples:

A person is on a spending spree and enjoying themselves with the purchases they make and thinking the bill will vanish. The thoughts that are running through their mind on how much they need and deserve the luxurious items without taking the time to create the funds to purchase them.

Another scenario is not letting anyone know of the comings and goings all day and night. The expectation is to be fed and have a roof over their head that is provided by someone else with no bills to pay and without contribution of any kind.

It is liberating to be treated like an adult and have the responsibilities and consequences that come along with graduating from childhood. The work and the successes that follow will bring inner peace and happiness.

USE VISION AND INTENTION WITH PURPOSE AND PLANNING

Starting with ONE problem increases the chances of obtaining a solution to get what you want. Many get discouraged if too much change is taken on all at once. Prevent being mentally overwhelmed before it starts. Overhauling many systems and structure too soon is a recipe for disaster. Maintaining routines by having discipline is extremely helpful and will save you from unnecessary failures.

Consistency Builds to Success

Doing something day in and day out even when it is tough is like exercise where you strengthen over time. This daily manna will become a lifeline so when the emergency or hard decision comes you will be ready to make it through.

Think of yourself sitting on the white sands of a peaceful beach and you know a violent storm is coming. Would you sit there and let the crashing waters come slap you in the face and take the beating? or would you become knowledgeable to know how to get out of the way by asking questions on the ways you can move forward. Your feelings of optimism and finding new ways to have solutions to the problems you are facing will become a way of life. Even though you may be wondering how this could be.

When to give and when to ask and receive help will be easier. Your stamina increases over time and before you know it you are achieving what you set out to do. Become a person of action.

GO LIVE WHAT YOU LEARN

Stay out of feast or famine mode by taking a step in the right direction. Consider an intersection and the four directions that lead to the same location is like solutions. There can be more than one right way that can offer relief and improvement. When you have the knowledge to make informed decisions and be responsible that you will accept the consequences that follow this can be freeing. Choice is the key!

There is a saying where there can be too much of a good thing. The same principle can apply to too little. Sunlight is an example of this where overdoing leads to sunburn and a certain amount of light is needed for optimum health. Find that sweet spot for effective and maximum performance. At first give yourself a range for success while you are learning and tweak along the way. Progress involves motion and momentum.

Living with optimism and temperance to have perspective that all things work for good are wonderful qualities to seek. What you are going through will become a gift to you one day with the lessons learned. Treasure the gifts of knowledge and wisdom that provide miracles when put to use.

Here is a wise quote.

"Only a fool learns from his own mistakes. The wise man learns from the mistakes of others."

Otto Von Bismarck

INVEST IN LEARNING

There was a dear family member that heard what was spent and said I could have had a college degree for that amount of money. What I wanted was a different kind of education than one in a traditional school setting. Seek out quality.

Looking back, what was very clear to me in my goals, was vague for others who were glad to help me if they only understood how. If you find this to be the case for you, take a deep breath and with patience the clarity will come. Over time you will be able to learn the skill of articulating your needs and wants.

Smiling comes to mind, as the first appointment with a mentor is remembered. Common questions are "What do you want more of?" Continued inner peace was one of the first replies. It's a bit puzzling for a guide to know how to measure results on the intangible. At first it was hard and embarrassing to feel like I was expressing what I wanted and getting feedback to be more specific when I thought I already was. Think of a toddler and their first words when they want something and it turns to tears and tantrums. The frustration is real as the little one tries to communicate.

If you feel like this is the case with you, repeat phrases to yourself such as "Hang in there", "The price is worth the wait", "I am Golden", "Sooner or later someone will understand".

HIRE A MENTOR/COACH

When it comes to a mentor/coach find someone who has already traveled the path and accomplished what you are seeking. Someone who is safe and can be trusted. They are committed to let you discover and explore your own transformation. By their example you know the small and simple steps to take as they walk WITH you.

Your time and energy will be saved as you are given insights to what you are blind to. Calendar the time when you will report back on how you are doing. When you meet together it is uplifting and edifying as you are asked to keep your commitments and stay accountable. Having someone who can give you appropriate correction and encouragement as needed is a gift.

Another tip to use if you are feeling buried under and over committed is to say "No" many more times than you say "Yes" without regret or apology. The sooner you make a decision and keep out of limbo land the better. This helps you maintain clarity and from being mentally overwhelmed. Focus and increased energy will also become your enthusiastic companion when you do this.

People around you will start to notice and take note. Write the feedback down and then you will see your strengths and progress too. Every ONE person will always become stronger with EVERYONE uplifted and united in a common cause that lifts others to be the best they can be. Some of these suggestions may sound too easy.

Try Simple, Simple, Simple and see if this is your key to Success!

Action steps

*What type of education are you seeking?

*Who would be a good teacher and support team and what qualities do they have?

*When will you ask mentor/someone to help you and with what?

*Will they encourage you in your dreams to help them come into reality?

*List experiences when you reached out and communicated and connected with someone that really listened and understood you. (Hint: this person would make a great coach or friend)

*If you are asking for more of something are you able to take care of what you have now?

Tips for the caregiver

*Keep a watchful eye and stand back far enough so your loved one has air to breathe and move forward with decisions when they are capable. Trust them when possible.

If you are working with someone fresh out of a hospitalization this is really difficult. Say a lot of prayers and the best care may end up coming from those who are unfamiliar with the past history and can keep emotions out of the decisions.

In the midst of the trial stay objective. Step in only when asked and is necessary for safety. Allow them to make mistakes and failures and learn from them. Even when they have a mental illness diagnosis let them explore what they can do for themselves. Doing too much for them can be a real pitfall.

*Have simple written rules and structure in place and follow through by doing what you say you will. This may be harder at first. Mental illness is not a free pass for them to do whatever they want. Keeping them responsible can be a challenge and is the loving way in the end.

*Ask good questions from what you are observing and make sure they are wanting suggestions. Here are some examples you could ask. "Who were you able to see today?" "What was a good thing that happened and what was something you would have liked to be better?" "Did you work?" What successes have you had?" These "kind of questions" will flow when you have a good relationship over time. Have an emotional bank account of deposits so when you need take a stand on the hard stuff that may require some withdrawals.

CHAPTER 7

THE GIFT OF HEALING THROUGH FORGIVENESS

Would you like to save time, feelings, and energy? There is a difference between learning from the past and living in it. Face your challenges and trials head on to decide what you can change and what to accept.

Preventing misunderstandings is much easier than resolving them. You'll be spinning your wheels if you start blaming, shaming, and pointing fingers. Resist the pitfalls of being tempted to focus on the errors of others, unkind acts towards you, or the rejection you are being subjected to.

If you end up taking a couple steps back make sure you are taking more steps forward then backwards. Leaving the judgment to God without taking things personal and giving each other the benefit of the doubt will save you from a lot of turmoil inside and out. Let yourself go to the space of love and forgiveness and your path of progress will be smoother and happier all around.

An example of this would be if someone is massively losing blood and bleeding to death you would get to work with the procedures that would be lifesaving. Just standing over the individual and talking about the past of the who done it's, would have, could have, should have, is a waste of time and time is a gift that we all have equal amounts of.

You are heading into a world of mystery and unknowns that can leave you with hurt feelings and an aching heart if you play the blame and regret game. Searching this way serves no one and can lead to a death spiral that is dark and becomes a big black bottomless pit. You will be ending up with more questions than what you started with. More than likely the conclusions will be speculation at best. Save yourself from dead ends.

Release yourself from the past quickly and start going the right direction as you look for what is going well in your life. My degree has been in the college of hard knocks and be assured the falling down and the getting up has been a great teacher.

Addressing the trials and afflictions with optimism along with the good times, keeps life real. We are all human and subject to errors and wrongs that are made by ourselves or others. Remember to not blame yourself either and let the one who is making bad choices carry their own burdens.

SILENCE IS NOT ALWAYS GOLDEN. Facing hard experiences will be harder at first but easier in the end. If you stuff feelings inside, hiding, or ignoring that the emotion is there will start creating a LIVE volcano inside of you. It becomes a matter of WHEN instead of IF the volcano will erupt.

Keep in mind there are some painful situations that can be blocked out of a person's memory. It's amazing how the brain protects us to stay safe. There may come a point when memories surface from an experience that you are having now that triggers the past. This is when working with someone who is trained and skilled is important and they can help you unravel the two separate issues of sexual abuse or past traumas is influencing the mental illness. They can be two separate issues.

Again, it is important to understand someone who is skilled in handling these types of situations that should be sought out. Once you recognize the problems, focus on ONE of them at a time.

Consider that silence is a choice with consequences as well. This is one tough lesson that I have learned and hope others can be spared this bucket load of tears. The decision to be quiet can be well intended when you are a peacemaker, yet it can have a ripple effect of damaging results.

What is your definition of forgiveness?

Sadly, there are people out there who take advantage of others. Most of the time someone saying sorry and restoration of what was lost is all that is necessary. In the cases where the laws are being broken and the offense is continuously repeated, this is when it is appropriate to step up and speak out to those in authority to enforce the law. Be a change agent and stop generations from the vicious cycle of innocent children and adults being taken advantage of.

MERCY CANNOT ROB JUSTICE

SILENCE or <u>Doing nothing</u> can leave a string of victims that can come from someone who sees they can get away with doing wrong. It is important to recognize the fallout of not saying anything. When it comes to your attention and you recognize the problem choose to come forward as what you remember loses accuracy over time. You are strong and can do what it takes.

Withholding information and giving someone a free pass to continue bad behavior creates a situation that will be difficult for the perpetrator too. What starts as a small problem turns into a hungry monster that continuously wants to be fed. Be brave and go to those who can help you take action, so all parties can be put on a path of healing. Coming out into the open is the forgiving thing to do for all those involved.

There are a few instances where allowing the legal system to take care of justice is necessary. Let them do the job of judgment. It requires courage to turn things over to those who have been given the authority. Make sure you are not taking the law into your own hands by being the judge and the jury. Society has created a justice system that even with imperfections, is better than carrying burdens yourself. Spiritual leaders are also ones who can help you with inner peace and have comfort as you bring wrongs into the light.

Resolving offenses sooner will always be better. When you get to that point "Let Go" as quickly as possible. You will be treading water for a long time or even worse drowning in sorrow if you stop forgiving. Even when you have had something taken from you that is irreplaceable in this life, hand it over to the legal system.

Know that one day whether it is in this life or in the eternities all wrongs will be made right in the hereafter. Pain and suffering is neutralized with forgiveness and love.

LOVE AND FORGIVENESS IS THE KEY TO HEALING

To determine how much of what you are going through is from mental illness versus what is from trauma can be pointless when there is no way to tell. Avoid these questions when they are UNPRODUCTIVE. What did I do to bring this upon myself? How did this happen? Where is God's love in this experience? Is sin the reason for this? If you are a caregiver and your relationship is being affected in a negative way with these types of question stay clear of them. You should have listened to me? Only take responsibility for what wrongs that are yours to make right.

FOCUS ON THE GOOD

Remembering it is great to give yourself permission to do something poorly while you are learning and growing. Forgive yourself as quickly as you forgive others.

BELIEVE IN SECOND CHANCES!

You have the ability inside of you to solve your own problems as you tap into your skills and learning. In other words, you can clean messes. Especially your own. We all make them. One way to think of this would be how your body digests food and eliminates waste naturally.

Our son in law was in a serious car accident. We all knew it was a miracle he was alive. When his children came to visit they would ask first thing if he had gone poo. It may seem a silly question to ask and yet when our bodies stop eliminating waste it becomes life threatening as it did in his case. The young children were so sweet and tears would come to my eyes as they would tell their Daddy not to die.

Asking such simple questions would lighten the mood as we found laughter and humor a great balm of sweet relief in a hard situation. Deal with the cards that you are dealt, make the best of the hand that is given you.

Forgiveness is great medicine to take care of your mental waste. The temporal, physical, and spiritual are all connected. Looking to God and trusting Him to be the Great Physician is the key, as we continue to do the best we can.

Forgiveness will allow illuminating love in the home. (literal and figuratively) Feel the love of God and let difficulties and challenges resolve on past traumas as quick as possible. (See sister's contribution) APPROPRIATE help when sought after and received will help you heal. Please consider there is no shame in seeking good council along with mighty faith and prayer.(See CPR for the soul contribution)

This lesson came home to my heart in a very real way as I sat in the courtroom with my son in law as he faced the man who had hurt him and that moment in time would have lasting consequences in this life not only for him but his family. (His contribution is at the end of this chapter along with the words he shared that day in court)

There wasn't a dry eye and the judge said the plus twenty years that he had been on the bench this was a first. The drunk driver apologized and read a letter and my son in law gave a great gift to himself to let his heart forgive the man who had trespassed against him and move forward with his life with faith knowing things work out especially when love and hope are the ultimate emotion that is carried into action.

Even though there was forgiveness the part the struck a chord with me was the legal counselors reminded us that there was more to the consequences than saying your sorry. Mercy could not be at the expense of justice. Really both families had been hurt and the Mother of the son who had caused so much pain cried in my arms. Each one of us had our own cross to bear and learn how to manage what was ahead of us. It was at this time that I was grateful for the legal system making the best decision they could within the framework of the law. Being judge and jury would have been unbearable.

Your attitude is different than your circumstance so chose to move forward with faith and forgive.

Action steps

*Write down the definition of forgiveness?

*Do you have a mess to clean up? If so with who? What? Commit to when you will take care of it.

*What did you learn? What can you let go of?

Contribution-Care giver-Sister

My sister Bonnie:

Her journey of healing after sexual abuse and mental illness

My sister and I have NEVER fought. I wonder how many siblings can boast that? It may be because there is more than a decade difference in age, or I would like to think that she is simply an angel. She is the oldest and I am in the middle of the ten children. As the oldest, she was like a second mother. To this day, I can always count on her support for important events and whenever I host family gatherings, she will always be found helping in the kitchen with clean up.

When I was young, I looked up to my sister in every way – she was beautiful and constantly dated (ask her how many times she went to Star Wars with different guys), was an honors student, and was genuinely kind. I had no idea she suffered in any way.

The sexual abuse she endured as a child had not been revealed and the struggle with depression and mental illness did not manifest outwardly until she was married with young children at home.

Feelings buried alive never die and hers erupted like a volcano. Where she had always been fiercely independent and service oriented, she now needed help during a complete collapse. This is one of those times that I am ever so grateful for a large family. Her kids were cared for and Bonnie was cared for day and night. We loved her. We prayed for her. We wondered if the Bonnie we knew would ever return. Unfortunately, it would be quite a bit later before she would get professional services because we didn't trust -shrinks and I think my grandma worried they would lock her up in a state institution and never let her out.

The other unfortunate thing was that I was told not to tell anyone about Bonnie and her condition. This was my introduction in dealing with mental health. I never knew until Bonnie's breakdown. It was one of those stay in the closet things.

Bonnie did get better. For a while. Years even. Grandma wasn't able to help anymore but others stepped in and again cared for Bonnie around the clock. I flew in from out of state to assist. She was reliving some of the horrors of her abuse in a mentally altered state and it was heartbreaking to witness. For all the people out there, who think abuse is no big deal, suck it up and get over it, you haven't a clue how damaging the trauma from abuse is on the victim. Her feelings that had been buried for a lifetime surfaced and the pain was immense. She could not bury them any longer. She would scream "Don't touch me! Leave me alone!" in a childlike state. She trusted no one in her paranoia. Sleep would not come for weeks.

Over the course of years, our family softened to the idea of getting medical intervention and Bonnie was hospitalized and medicated. The medications did seem to bring her back to her senses faster. We discovered that the medical professionals were helpful but can be very difficult to access. Their patient loads are so heavy it is difficult to get help in less than a month's time. Hospital beds for the mentally ill are often full, and the cost of the stays can bankrupt families.

Bonnie also realized she needed help and tried everything she could think of to have healing in her life. She met with her ecclesiastical leaders and relied on her faith. She met with counselors, medical doctors, psychiatrists and psychologists. She tried to find the right balance of meds, sleep, stress, diet and exercise. She signed up with mentors and coaches to help her change the dialogue in her head. She spent intensive years trying to figure herself out. Once she discovered balance in her life, she made it a mission to share her experience and try and help others so they too can have peace.

I am grateful to her for Bonnie nver giving up. That she has been able find healing and balance and even if she finds herself out of balance, she now has a tool box of ways to help herself mend. Love you Sis!

~*Contribution Son-In-Law*~

As I drive this road each morning I contemplate on the marks in the ground which almost became the resting spot of a sidewalk wreath. This morning I had a very poignant thought that became the inspiration for the following message. I wish I could express it as I talked, but my tears would stop me from finishing. Please take a few minutes to read and ponder.

A year ago, I had the privilege of celebrating Easter focused on the spiritual message of Christ and his love for his brothers and sisters as I recovered in a hospital bed. I have learned so many lessons as I have suffered through physical pain and spiritual anguish. I have come to know and believe in Christ at a level that has changed my life and forever shapes me as a man, father, spouse, brother, friend, and example.

"I stand all amazed at the love Jesus offers me. Confused at the grace that so fully he proffers me. I tremble to know that for me he was crucified.

That for me, a sinner, he suffered, he bled and
died. Oh, it is wonderful that he should care for me

Enough to die for me! Oh, it is wonderful,
wonderful to me!" (Lds hymn 193)

The night of my accident exactly a year ago is still
a blur; however, I vividly still remember the peace
and love of Christ and God that I felt as I awoke
and regained consciousness. This feeling was so
strong and powerful and encompassed my heart.
Oh I wish I could describe how deep, soul freeing,
and powerful Gods love for you feels as death door
knocks.

I strive each day to stay close to this feeling. It
changed me. I plead for all who have witnessed the
miracle [of] my life to stay close to God. Believe
in him. Believe and live your lives loving and
forgiving others. The memories and love you
shared with others during this life will fast forward
in the present as you stand at the door of death. I
am privileged to continue to make memories and
be there as a friend for countless others while I
fulfill the new mission God has for me.

I am doing very well. My physical infirmities are healing, but more importantly my soul is becoming more Christlike. I have shed tears over the year hoping I can be an example of his love and help you to feel his love. I commit to do my part.

God lives. God loves. Jesus is the Christ and will come again. I can't wait to cry at his feet and say Thank you, Thank you, Thank you!!! I LOVE YOU! I LOVE YOU! I LOVE YOU!

Easter has forever been changed for me. We will all rise again with our Lord, Master, Friend, Redeemer, and Savior. He suffered, died, and was resurrected for YOU!

(The Story Continues)

Sentencing is over and am able to move on to next chapter in life. Here are the remarks I felt Impressed to share at [the court] sentencing.

Six months ago the car wreck I was involved in changed my life dramatically.

The worries and pain of my physical infirmities will be with me and my family for the rest of my mortal life. The financial burden that my family may face due to my early potential death may become a challenge. The stress and impact on my wife, children, and family the past few months are hard to quantify let alone put into words.

With these challenges it would be very easy to be bitter and vindictive against [this impaired man]. However, from the moment I came to full consciousness a few days after the accident I have felt a different spirit. I found a spirit of gratitude to be alive. I found Jesus Christ's spirit of love and look forward to being with family, friends, and a community that loved me for a few more years. But, Most importantly I found the spirit of Christ's atonement and mercy in forgiving me of my sins and my ability to forgive [this man] for causing some setbacks.

I was humbled by the many prayers offered in my and [the impaired driver's] behalf. My children's and wife's prayers for his recovery touched my heart. We continue to pray for his ability to recovery from alcoholism and pray that he will find peace in following the Lord.

My recovery has been a miracle. The events of that night and the participants placed in the experience were not there by coincidence . I stand before the court this day to boldly exclaim that Heavenly Father, Jesus Christ, and the Holy Spirit are real. There is life after death. The peace and love in that location are worth living a good life on the earth. My life's mission is to be an example of Christs love for all others to feel. I will go to my grave helping others know that they are unconditionally loved by the Lord.

[Looking to the drunk driver:] Please take this time of temporary setback and put your life in the ultimate direction you want it to go. Honor the men and women in your life that love you and prove to them that you can live a life full of love and compassion.

Thanks to my family members, doctors, and nurses who spent many nights tending to me and helping me recover from the many injuries. Finally thanks to my dear wife who has been by my side through this entire experience. I will be forever indebted to her and the example she set for our beautiful three children. Her name will be honored and revered for eternity.

CHAPTER 8

THE GIFT OF SERVICE AND GRATITUDE

THE GIFT OF SERVICE AND GRATITUDE

Different perspectives are important as you reflect what you can offer that is valuable. Visualize a day when you are out talking with people. Do you notice any common feedback? If you notice a theme from several different people they may be recognizing some things you need to pay attention to for improvement. You also can receive insights about your talents and gifts and this will help you know how to serve.

There is another dimension that comes with intuition and you will find yourself being at the right place with the right person, at the right time. This has been the case with me as miracles have happened on a daily basis. Children are especially in tune as you show them how to follow your footsteps. You can learn from them too.

One time my grandson and I were able to go into an Alzheimer's unit. At first he was hesitant and afraid but as the residents begged for his attention the smiles and laughter began for all of us. It was contagious and fun.

The story of the Starfish hung on the wall there and we knew our visit made a difference to each person. You know the story-

Once a starfish washed up on the beach that would soon die in the hot sun. There was one little child who threw a few back but could, of course, not save them all. When asked why he tried because he could never make a difference to them all, he picked one up, threw it into the ocean and said, "I made a difference to that one." Service starts with ONE and be full of GRATITUDE for the opportunity to do so.

One time I saw a little baby being helped with a major skin problem. While I was sitting there the question came to my mind if perhaps this would be a day when I would be completely healed.

There was a tender visual that came to my mind of the Savior wearing ALL the thorns as a crown was placed on his head. His reply to me is you have only had to carry ONE. This put what I was going through in life in a beautiful perspective of gratitude. The answer was NO and that not ALL symptoms would be removed, however the peace and comfort in my heart was there in all the ways that matter. Paul in the scriptures asked for a thorn to removed and it wasn't. Over the years it is nice to see the support that has always been there from angels on earth and in heaven to lighten the load and burdens. You can choose to be bitter or better. The ALL-IN gratitude is finding the blessing in the bad, the ugly, and the good.

When you are in an accident or a mess how do you react to them? You will notice a shift in your attitude if you stay positive in a negative situation and in a few short weeks with consistent gratitude you will feel 100% better than you did before.

WRITE WHAT YOUR GRATEFUL FOR AND YOU WILL START TO SEE WAYS TO HELP YOURSELF

Life is like a tapestry with the dark and light threads woven in between. Or a canvas with a mixture of colors with contrasting paint that adds richness and fullness to the work of art. Each person is a masterpiece of the master artist. Over time each thread becomes meaningful and appreciated for the contribution that is being made to give depth and beauty to all who see.

Let it be said by others that your reputation is one of integrity and honesty for those who want to know more about you. Most importantly are the promises that you make and keep to yourself. As Shakespeare said, "To thine own self be true."

WRITE your own story of progress. Any other way the facts become embellished into fiction and folklore. Have courage in knowing that your message has much to offer. Our legacy is what we leave for our posterity. Share what you learned from challenges and how you overcame them.

Teach how you grew as a person and found solutions. How you worked to experience the triumphs. Remember the ride of life only comes around once and you get to decide what kind of ride it will be. Perhaps the sweetest victories are the ones you work the hardest to have!

Keep a tablet handy at bedside and as you go about your day to record impressions. Pay attention to your dreams. When you wake up ask yourself to remember what your subconscious and unconscious mind was trying to teach you in your sleep.

RECORD SUCCESSES AND CELEBRATE

Many times, it's easier to know how to celebrate big but do you know ways to celebrate simple and small too? Doing something like going out in the sun, breathing deeply, or throwing a snowball takes only a few moments and a great stress reliever. The key is choosing what you can do that will bring JOY right NOW.

After being able to do a step towards your goal be sure to thank God who is the giver of all good gifts. Be grateful for what you have as you ask to receive more. Your beautiful body and mind is the vehicle that provides the opportunity to-CRY, SMILE, LAUGH, AND HAVE A SENSE OF HUMOR, EAT, SLEEP, AND LIVE!

Action Steps-

*Each day pray and LISTEN to who you can assist. WRITE the name down on your daily list.

*Set a reminder (alarm to help you remember when you will connect with the person you were thinking about.

* Start and end your day with thinking of five things you are thankful for. Stretch yourself into recognizing what is unusual and out of the ordinary that blesses your life.

*Keep a gratitude journal of what you have learned for yourself and your posterity.

*Help with grief can be found by asking funeral directors if they know of any classes or groups that you can connect with. Literature can be found there too. Senior community centers and libraries are good places for resources as well.

Contribution-Caregiver-Family-Father-Husband

While actively involved in so many various events and activities and sensing the importance of taking the time to remedy signs of potential disasters coming forth. These significant and important activities at the time included the raising of five beautiful daughters, full time work, full and overtime school, and working a major research and marketing project.

Along with this additional project required a licensing to marketing rights with infomercials covering Us and South America markets, requiring a large deposit already made and mortgaging our home. The sudden death of the project manager involved in this project also complicated life.

Because of my busy life style at this time, I started to notice important abnormalities in my wife's unusual behavior, which included sleepless nights, stressful, adaptation, lack of eating, intense and sporadic statements about news articles such as words stating "the world is in so much turmoil", along with date's, memorabilia, and various phrases of words associated with world problems that she emphasized that was abnormal to her prior behavior. This included topics such as war and especially topics included with religion, epic events, connections, and exaggerations as to why,

*when, how soon, and where and these events are
happening.*
Total chaos and turmoil ensued.

*So, arrangements were made for the two of us to
stay at the Grandmothers to get some peace of
mind. This provided a way to have her reluctant
Grandmother to assist in getting my wife to see a
Doctor for an evaluation. With this unusual wife's
behavior, all pending events including school,
work, marketing, research, etc. was suddenly
scrapped. This also included the kids going to
lessons up to thirty miles away, dancing, music,
gymnastics, and still getting the kids off to school
was quite a juggling act. This abnormal and
awkward behavior was indeed challenging and
was turning our family world upside down.*

*It was at this moment in time my real character
was being challenged. After the interviewing and
evaluating Doctor completed his verbal interview
with my wife and grandmother, there was a brief
but shocking interview with me. My wife and
Grandmother went to a side room. This allowed
the Doctor to visit with me alone. This is what I
remember him stating, "So, there is a lot going on
in your home" and "YOU! "are the major cause
of this disconnect of realty your wife is going
through."*
*"**BAM**"!! This was indeed a "BLOW" and red
dagger spear to my "HEART". In my mind I*

rehearsed, Yes, I wasn't the perfect husband in the world", we as a couple don't agree on a lot of things, but to me that is just part of marriage in my mind. How preposterous I thought, "I would never want to hurt my wife in any way physically or mentally".I had been so involved in so many activities that I had somewhat, you might say dislodged or disconnected myself to those most important matters that bind and seal family relationships through sincere communication efforts vital to supporting one another. Togetherness is so much more valuable to me than all the outside projects that pull in the opposite direction of strengthening families."I am presently a little teary-eyed stating this". For the Doctor to state that I was the cause of the situation was very detrimental to me. My understanding and willingness to accept that reality didn't hit me the hardest at that moment, but a little latter.

My wife and I stayed at her grandmothers while our children were cared for by others. Grandmother had great intentions and while stating and repeating, "don't ever again enter into the Doctor's path again. "We can handle these family matters ourselves" she stated: I respected Grandmothers wishes and new she meant well. She was very set in her ways. Very direct in her persuasive and powerful statements and expressing her opinions in a passionate and penetrating way. "Loved Her". "oops", "Teary-eyed again"

Very shortly after the Doctor's visit, my wife's eating disorder was now fully kicking in. What I mean to say is she just didn't want to eat. I was, in my mind, trying every way I could think of to get her to eat. Not only food, but also trying various sorts of herbs, vitamins, fruits, vegie's, anything of good report. Memories of Grandmother stating, "do not involve the medical doctors". This statement was constantly recycling in my head. I seriously wrestled with this differing opinion.

My wife just didn't want to eat without almost forcing her to. The evaluation Doctor prescribed sleeping meds which seemed to backfire and cause just the opposite reaction of what it was meant for which caused her to not sleep. Sleep segments in the middle of the night seemed to only last in segments of only about two hours. We, as her immediate family, assisted as much as possible, singing together, using soft music, prayers, and tons of faith. This continued to take its toll on myself as well as the family. My dear spouse had, a lack of cooperativeness, increased rebelliousness, and unawareness of reality magnified in her lack of ability to communicate. She also had distorted, confusing, disconnected body motions, and disjointed words. Phrases were hidden and continued to worsen and increase, for example, "Why do this", rather than "why are you doing this". Or "me do it", rather than "can I do it?" It would have been better to have used smoke signals or sign language to communicate with her, than to communicate with her normally.

To also assist in handling the situation, we put her in an enlarged walk in closet in the basement with the assistance of family members twenty-four-seven. This was due to her body motions being sporadic and moving in obstinate and possible obstructive mannerisms without realizing possible endangerment to herself. Her weight loss quickly went down from 160 pounds to 119 pounds within a few short days. Our continued thoughts were that she would be ok as soon as she would start eating and sleeping right.

Reflecting upon Grandmothers words of wisdom, helped us to come up with a plan of action to where we could take care of her until we felt she might recover. The large closet which was more like a small comfortable room, no windows, with a mattress and pillows placed on the floor and along the walls, providing a safe zone for everyone assisting.

After nearly two weeks of relying on our own endeavors and not understanding the emergency situation we were in, we took my wife to an institution nearly 60 miles away for an injection

161

that was supposed to have helped turn her return to normal. This didn't seem to help. Also, while trying to manhandle her upstairs at the home, it took at least three or four persons to assist in persuading her to stand up and move cooperatively. A neighbor came over, (and he, being diabetic), understood the mental condition and physical nature of the situation going on, and stated: "You must get her immediately to the hospital". "This is an emergency and very dangerous to her health and well-being". Like a flash of lightning, we quickly manhandled her to the car, (not easily done), and immediately took her off to the hospital at this time. We had to sign my wife into the hospital psych ward. Upon signing my wife in, we didn't realize that our rights and hers, were taken away. What I mean to say, is that the hospital allows you to sign a patient into the psych ward, however, does not allow you to withdraw them out of the psych ward at your convenience.

It was after this event that I personally had my reawakening. Due to the wife gone and the hospital staff stating that she may be there six months to two years without allowing me to decide when to have her released. It would be up to the hospital to make that determination at their discretion with this unforeseen information, it was like a light bulb that went on in my head. I mean to say a dark light bulb. I realized some brutal facts,

"The possibility of her not regaining normal function again". The Children, The Family, work, and a purpose in life.

With this aftermath upon me and while at work, trying with my head and heart to understand the possibility of what I may have assisted in causing, I was overwhelmed with this reality. The love that I had for my wife, her grandmother, my wonderful children and my wife's family. These thoughts suddenly took a huge toll on me mentally, physically, and were financially disturbing. For a brief moment, I even had thoughts of wanting to leave the planet. I couldn't take it anymore. Thoughts of anguish, torment and destructiveness were occupying and conquering my mind. Yes, I thought in that short, quick moment, it's time to find a way out of this world.

However, suddenly good thoughts of positive and productive core values floated to the surface within my soul. I was able to get a hold of my sickening adversarial thoughts and realizing a higher level of understanding to my true calling as a Father, provider, husband, and most of all, a dedicated Husband and Father. This focus led quickly to clarification of my responsibilities and accountability. As a Father, I knew I must be committed to being available to meet the challenges, trails, obstacle's, and pressures life presents. No one say's it's going to be easy, but it will be worth it.

Within 10 Days in the hospital the tables turned. Due to the modern meds etc. and professional help and assistance, the sweetest kind loving Wife and Mother was on her way back to reality.

Oh, what joy!

Home sweet home shortly afterward (at the home of my in-laws) another very special person came. He had been a teacher for the blind and deaf for over 30 years. He had a most remarkable understanding of the mind, how it functions, processes, and understands. With his special experience and ability, he was able to assist my wife with thought patterns in a way to have her mentally respond with quick, amazing perceptive responses and understanding. It was simply remarkable. He also stated that "in the future this will be a blessing for her to share and assist others in similar situations".

A few years later a similar situation arose. This time, my wife was able to recognize the patterns, feelings and direction she was going into. Because of this her preparation, she was able to have a much more self-understanding which gave her the ability to admit herself into the hospital to get proper medication and help. Again, this was due to her determination, sole searching, and preparation as well as her constant seeking to assist in preventing a re-occurrence. By her admitting herself into the hospital, gave her the mental capacity and ability to check herself IN and OUT on her own when prepared and ready to go. By my wife doing this, took the responsibility and authority off of me as well as the hospital workers for discharge approval. This was so much smother and easier than the first time when I felt accountable and yet even then could not approve her discharge.

So, when you have the thoughts it's time to get off the planet, you have the freedom, right and privilege to change thoughts to overcome and kick the dark light bulb out, realizing there is help and hope ahead, and replace the darkness with a BRILLIANT INNER LIGHT WITHIN

From the Family today, consisting of 7 children and 16 grandchildren we thank all those involved. Remarkable outcomes have been priceless. Special thanks to the Blind and Deaf teacher and instructor, Robert Fletcher, his optimistic input and assistance, and also the qualified Medical Teams. We are so appreciative for the learning experiences and strengthening of a most beautiful family. These experiences have prepared our family with the importance of seeking proper professional help.

CHAPTER 9

THE GIFT OF COMMUNICATION

THE GIFT OF COMMUNICATION

Surround yourself with those who lift you up!
Counsel and work together as a team!

Research is finding out how important
socialization is to our health and well-being. There
have been studies of little babies whose basic
needs of being fed and clean without being
cuddled and touched lead to failure to thrive.
Tender care and touch is essential.

Along with the physical and being with someone
in person is being able to have healthy
Communication and Connection with them. Have
you ever been on the phone trying to make a
connection and feeling like no one is listening on
the other side of the line? Let both sides be heard
and edified.

It's like an onion, you peel it a layer at a time. One
problem at a time. By trying one solution at a time,
and one success they are seeing with each step
they are taking forward. You will receive many
ideas from those around you and it is up to you to
decide the ONE principle (that's the layer) and the
first action step to begin with. Where you are right
now is what counts and how you will know where
to begin. Speak up. Get some ideas and then start.
Put one foot in front of the other and before you
know it you will be amazed how far you have

come. Realize that some layers will require some trial and error. This is when healthy tears might be appropriate as you re-calibrate and get yourself on the path of progression again. Crying can be healthy and bring relief.

Brainstorming with other people can help you discover options and solutions so taking the hits of the big waves from the storms of life will be much easier. Have an action partner you can talk to. Imagine this twosome as being a circle of synergy that evenly flows as each freely gives and receives. Be open enough that the person you trust can be honest with you. It would be like a door handle and you need both sides for it to fill its function and purpose. Come to a meeting of the minds and a true connection. No one is sacrificing when you identify and create common ground together that satisfies the needs and wants of both.

Each one of the partnership is equal. One way to know if you have the give and receive going full circle is to see if you can accept a compliment as graciously as you can give it. When this is smooth you have a WIN/WIN situation that is richly rewarding.

Helen Keller is a lady who exemplified how you can feel and then learn to express yourself appropriately.

The story of this blind child trying to express herself with frustration has had a familiar ring to it for me as the time approached to face these unstable states of mind and how there was acting out that was very difficult for others to know what to do. Thankfully the family did not enable me and hung in there under these trying times until professionals came on board to assist in unraveling the conversations to get to the truths.

There were some variables of the past where I thought I was serving others best by staying silent. It was a rude awakening to find out how it would have been much better to come forward to the right people in appropriate ways and speak up. What I have come to realize is communication is a skill.

When the lines of connection are shut down it can wreak all kinds of havoc inside an individual. It's understandable how aggravating it would have been for Helen to have such a brilliant mind and not be able to hear, speak, or see. Perhaps you feel this way when trying to talk about what you want. Keep going and set a daily goal to find someone who will listen to you and keep the conversation positive.

One of the ways to learn to not bite the hand that feeds you, is the principle of LISTENING IN THREES. This may come from someone talking to you or what you read, see, or hear. If this comes up three times decide to take heed and PAY ATTENTION! Have some curiosity as to why this is coming up. Go ahead and ponder if this is an area you will want to improve.

No one is perfect and be able to be flexible enough to try new ways that will benefit you and bless those you interact with. A highly successful business mentor shared the scariest person to work with is the one who thinks they know it all, when they really don't. No one knows everything. Be careful with how many people and how much information you gather to stay out of confusion and paralysis by analysis. Documenting what is said and what is important will help you keep things accurate. Misunderstandings can be readily resolved when what you have learned is fresh and written down. Waiting too long and exercising extreme caution to avoid a mistake or seeking the perfect answer will slow you down. Trial and error can work out too.

Using intention and being specific as you can on what you want can help the caregivers be able see what is reasonable and possible. For those on your team this will require a lot of faith and trust in you too. Time may be necessary to process what opportunities are best, so ask when it can be brought up again so you can come to a resolution.

Realize a lot of change all at once will take you longer. If you are comparing results to another, STOP. That's a winding road of detours you are going to be so glad to quit taking. If you are going to compare let it be your own progress! The consequences will follow regardless. Are you ready to accept the results? Report back with accountability as you work with others and by learning healthy communication skills, you will go a long way using this formula.

Speak up and Keep your dreams alive!

What I found is how many people really wanted to help me if they only knew how. Keep going back and forth with each other until the question of what is wanted is clear. Let others help you with this. Be ready to answer questions such as what is the top two things you want to accomplish? How is your moods and your stress? What are you doing to manage? Are you results what you want?
Pay attention to how you communicate with yourself and listen to the mental chatter. Is what you are saying about yourself in your head something you would say to someone else? Catch the negative words that put you in a downward spiral to a halt. Let what you hear be edifying and about how wonderful you are.

Mental illness can become life threatening if you quit paying attention to the details. By details this could mean lack of sleep, irritability, withdrawn, changes in behavior, etc. When someone is in a psychotic state of mind they are challenging as there can be several days and nights of no sleep, wandering off, undressing, no control of urine and bowel movements, a loss of appetite, weight loss, body organs shutting down, to name a few of the symptoms that can develop.

Extreme highs in mood are as life threatening as the lows and my mind had so many thoughts and actions that stopping to eat and take care of basic personal hygiene became unimportant. Talking was fast and hard for others to understand. These are danger zones to be aware of and stay far away from. Give permission for someone to take action if you have a 911 emergency.

The odds I was given almost twenty plus years ago was close to zero to live a normal life. In fact, institutionalization was suggested. Now hearing repetitively by family, friends, medical doctors and professionals that I am normal and not crazy and that is music to the ears.

You may be tempted to go through the past and wonder if you would have done something wrong to bring this trial upon yourself. When will this nightmare end? Is there anything I could have done to escape this affliction? The answer is probably not.

I'm a huge believer in the law of abundance, positive thinking, visualization and having goodness manifest in your life. In fact, my nickname from friends is "Polyanna". This name comes from a movie where the young girl would take every situation and make the best of it. Truth is we are subject to ailments in body and mind because we are human. You may hear others tell you to have more faith and pray more to be well. Even worse you are evil. Bad things can happen to great people. Life is Life and knowing when you brought this upon yourself versus when you are having a mortal experience can give peace of mind to know how to proceed. Be wise to who and what you listen to and get the help you need.

After the hospitalization, a great healer came into my life named Robert Fletcher. The knowledge he taught about the mind was a great comfort as my memory began to come back. Robert's uncle Harvey Fletcher was a friend with Albert Einstein and their family has blessed the world with many inventions in space, the hearing aid, and stereophonic sound. He is the founder of thought pattern management (TPM) and the techniques that are used give you the permission to unleash the power of your subconscious and unconscious mind to start the healing process within yourself.
Be persistent and forgiving to yourself and others. Triggers may come up. These can be words,

feelings, smells, thoughts, that set you up for looping into the past.

It was my opportunity to later be schooled and sit knee to knee with psychiatrists, neurologist, and other professionals in other fields who had heard of the successes of TPM and we learned how to talk gently to the mind and inner self to have amazing results.

When you catch onto these thoughts and the way the brain tries to keep safe then you can turn these patterns to be in a productive direction is really rewarding. This knowledge proved very valuable in my healing.

Ask yourself, "Who is in my circle of trust?" (This can be family friends, clergy, doctors, holistic practitioners, etc.) What can I talk to them about? When? Where? For how long? When will I report back the action steps I chose to take? Will they listen to my successes? Do you know ahead of time what is to be exchanged? (example-time for time, a trade, or exchange of money)

Teach others how to respond to you by using phrases such as…"Do I have permission to share"…"May I suggest"…" Is there anything I said that rang true for you"…"
BE ALL IN and give YOUR 100%!

The question to ask yourself is what are you willing to do about it?

When you have enough knowledge to begin now and know that **you GET TO go into the lab and GO TO WORK.** After the talk it is time to see yourself walking the talk, by taking action! COMMIT!

Yes, commit to who, what, when, and where. Often times the world gives a quick sell that leaves out the part of all work that is necessary to get from point A-Z. Learn to Pay the Price to get where you want to be.

Remember caregivers, using FORCE will backfire. Know when to let go. Say your prayers for the one you care about. Whatever steps your loved one takes backwards they will want to get out of the pain and in the end become stronger when they figure out how to move forward. Tough love may be necessary at times. The work of the process is what matters along with finding happiness as you go on your way.

Here is an example of family trying to shield me from bad memories and yet it became a relief to me once I saw the situation for what it really was. Let the light into the traumatic memory and let the monster go. When my health returned I faced the dreaded closet by literally going into it and laughing to find it was just that…a big walk in closet.

The gaps in memory might be significant if you have had deep psychosis. I would compare it to being in a black hole and not being able to know the specifics of how to climb out into the light. I found time to be non-existent and the days and nights all mixed into one. Fill the dark feelings with what was real by asking those in your circle of trust to help you remember. What you find out may be different than what you want to hear, such as you had a problem.

I remember having some great conversations with my brother in law that were completely coherent. Unfortunately for him they came in the middle of the night. He would comment, "Oh you're back". This left me thinking where had I been? It was shocking to me to realize days and nights had passed and I had no awareness of that at all. My church leaders advised the family that along with faith and blessings it was encouraged that I be taken to the emergency room as the situation was getting critical. This physical and mental illness affected the spiritual too. In the scriptures Christ was asked who sinned the child or the parents and the reply was neither. If mental illness is something that you deal with remember YOU ARE NOT EVIL! When you are mentally stable be careful what you attribute to the adversary. In fact, my recommendation is to leave the devil out of it and treat this illness like any other. Often when there are mental symptoms there are physical reasons as to why the thoughts are being affected that need to be addressed. When I began to be more stable and came home from the hospital feelings of guilt would come up and this is when the prayers and help from loved ones and church leaders helped.

It's interesting how the media reports a crime and contributes what happened to mental illness. How often have you heard a reporter say this criminal did this because he has eye problems, diabetes, high blood pressure, or some other physical ailment? Most people with a mental illness diagnosis are not going to commit a violent crime. If this was the case there would be many more incidents than there are now if it correlated to how many have a diagnosis. Let's put a halt to the idea and actions in society that are perpetuating stigmas and preventing those who want to receive care from getting it. Start a movement by being the one who is an advocate for those who are in need of compassion.

Action Steps

*What decisions are you making right now? Decide WHEN you will say yes or no.

*Really get down on your knees and pray and ask and listen for the answer.

* Who can you confide in, where there is uplifting two-way communication?

*Selectively pick the best of the best counsel and form ONE plan.

*Journal a time when you shared what you learned from successes AND a failure.

*Write down an unexpected kindness or reward that you received in word or deed.

Tips for caregivers

Caregivers have set rules with healthy boundaries that will offer your loved one ways to have confidence, trust, and courage within themselves.

CHAPTER 10

⏳ THE GIFT OF TIME AND MONEY $$$

MONEY IS GOOD WHEN IT IS USED TO BLESS YOURSELF AND OTHERS

A common avoided subject is the five-letter word-MONEY.

You may think that the TIME and MONEY to go to doctor appointments is too expensive and not worth it. Consider the alternatives. **Intensive care units or planning a funeral is worse.**

How much is doing nothing costing you?

Know that- **Silence has a price too!**

The sooner you invest in yourself by speaking up to receive help in a timely way the better.
Money is neutral not evil. Like the sun shining on all, the evil and the good, the same applies with this finances.

When I went into a crisis this is when my quirks showed up. For me some of them were about time and money. Let me share an example of what I talked about in a psychotic state. The paranoia was real. One of those fears was that everyone was out to take all our money. If I heard anyone asking for money they were evil and not to be listened too. After a while that was pretty much anyone that was working to keep me safe and follow rules. Doctors, clergy, and close family and friends became a part of this delusion. When someone gets to this point, helping them will be much more difficult and expensive.

Again, prevention and having a plan in place will assist you to know what actions to take without hesitation. Whatever tasks your loved one does their disability will put them out of commission and leave you to pick up the slack. Make sure it is discussed and correlated when bills are due and how they are paid especially if the one who takes care of these matters becomes unable to do so. Keeping tabs on what each one does will make distributing the tasks to others easier so daily living is kept flowing with a minimal amount of disruptions as possible.

If you realize you are having difficulty investing in yourself you may have some strange thoughts coming to mind. These patterns may have developed while you were young. An example of this would be: if I am wealthy then my children will be spoiled and unproductive.
Whether you are poor or rich money can be misused. Often you hear strange things from those who have less about those who have more money or in reverse. This kind of pattern can be affecting you now without your awareness.

Blessings are much more easily recognized when you have the necessities. Even better is when you have enough and to spare. Having the means to financially provide jobs or serve in the community has wonderful benefits for the giver as well as the receiver. Think how hard it is to be happy when you are out in the cold with an empty stomach and no roof over your head.

Many of those who are homeless suffer from mental illness and are in need of compassion and guidance in knowing how to take care of themselves and stop the cycle. Can you be spiritual when you are hungry and downtrodden? The physical, mental, spiritual, emotional, and financial areas are all connected. When there is weakness in one area it can bleed into and affect the other parts of our lives.

I'd like to share a fun little story that happened about earning and handling money. It has proven to be a great learning tool and asset to me.

One day I was lying in bed mid-morning and awakened by my husband to come and talk to some people who were coming to buy a piece of furniture. My help was needed. I was really reluctant because my hair was a mess and I was still in my PJ's because of the long work hours I had the day before. In my mind I was totally convincing myself I deserved the rest. The mood was totally lacking in enthusiasm and the thoughts in my head were screaming, "Stop. No. Not Now."

Thankfully I recognized this self- sabotage dialog and decided to put a halt to this inner grumbely voice. This was an excuse. My Grandma would say, "Get your rear and gear." In a few minutes my hair was brushed and I quickly changed.
A brief glance in the mirror discovered I was actually ok and found I looked nice enough to wear a smile and say hello.

A sweet surprise was in store. There were four lovely people of integrity that were there to buy a chair for a friend who had suffered a head injury. The connection of trust was quickly established as we got to know one another and found common ground through the artwork in our home and we talked about knowing the artist who did this book cover.

We talked and they tested the chair to see if it was going to work. It became clear this was a perfect fit for their friend and now time to close the deal.

The money was about to be exchanged when my husband asked them to give it to my wife and she will handle the money. This came as a surprise to me so when it was time to hold the cash I wrapped it up in my hand and didn't count it because they were people we had built a rapport with and trusted them.

A ten-dollar discount was discussed and they said, "Honey you keep that excess $10. We are glad to pay the asking price", which amounted to $250.

Later I was doing a meditation and had the book with the money in it sitting on my lap. I went to give half the money to my husband who was so kind to offer me all of the money from the sale. We discovered there were two $50's, two $20's and one $10. That's when the mystery began as it was clear that adds up to only $150.

I thought to myself, "Am I going crazy"? After searching high and low with my husband helping me I concluded I must have lost the $100. When I was asked if I counted the money with the buyers, I had to say "No".

Big financial lesson-

COUNT THE MONEY

It began to occur to me that if I went into a bank would they trust me and just hand over a stack of bills. The answer is obvious and clear when each one of you see the money out in the open there is a meeting of the minds that builds trust. Boy would I have been doing us all a favor if the money was handled in a professional way. Realizing this was my fault I was quick to adjusting so that I could be happy with only $150.

I'm glad I'm married to someone who likes to get to the bottom of things and following through by calling the man and asking if he had given me too much money. It was hilarious when he said "NO" and went on to say how he was an engineer and rarely made mistakes.

To his horror as he repeated back the denominations of the two 50's, and two $20's and one $10. He then realized he had made a mistake and was quick to apologize and put a check in the mail. Wow, the relief was great when I realized I hadn't lost my mind or the money and was so grateful to work with such honest people.

By pursuing this to the end it became an even higher level of exchange and a bigger win-win. If that call was not made I would have been happy with $150 but would always have wondered what had happened. I've also related this to conversations where we stop just before we really are about to get to know one another better. When a problem comes up and we hesitate and never pick up the phone to ask the questions and see if a best solution can be found, rather than settling with our own ideas, conclusions and outcomes.

Use due diligence to protect yourself from fraud. This is best done ahead of time when the heart and mind are clear. When you know you have covered your bases it makes it much easier to know what to do to avoid being ripped off when you are vulnerable. Stay accountable for what you chose to spend your money on will also benefit you when challenges come up and the results are different than what you hoped for.

An Italian proverb says-

"He that deceives me Once, it's his fault, twice it is my fault."

I've received calls from family and others asking if the money was worth spending over the many years. The answer is a resounding "Yes". One of the symptoms of not managing bipolar is spending too much, so this was a question I was glad that I was asked and able to answer. If you were going to have eye surgery would you trust someone with no education or experience with your valuable vision because they are less money? Every penny is a penny well spent when it comes to improving education and health.

Have you put a price tag on you? If you are waiting for the best deal you may be dragging things out and making life harder than necessary. when money becomes the #1 focus in your decisions. Become familiar with your insurance policies and have money set aside for prevention care so you are not shopping around for the best price when you want medical attention. It is a myth that healing is pain free. If you fall down and break a leg it is going to hurt as you receive treatments? Yes, healing hurts. Paul in the Bible asked the thorn in his side to be removed. It was left there and he learned how to manage it. When you get to this point of acceptance you will know you are in a good place of recovery.

After a season the fruits of my labor began to be noticed and the personal transformation was significant. Take a financial self-assessment and to evaluate where you are at now and how you can take the steps to be where you want to be in the future.

Action Steps

*Make an appointment today that is for maintenance and prevention for your mental and physical well-being.

*Now you are in a place of stability decide what you want to do to sustain this. (Ideas-doctor appointments, haircuts, massages, night out, an educational classes)

*What can you do to recognize your contribution and value?

*Are your unanswered questions being answered?

*Do you have a budget?

*Divide a paper in half and write possible risks and rewards. Then make a decision.
*How will you know when you've identified positive results?

Summary of Solutions
and Problems

PROBLEMS
*SILENCE
* Where to find good help?
* The cost of care and medicine
* Suicide
* Awareness from the loved one that they need help
*Misunderstandings that come up by taking the sickness personal (This includes the one with the diagnosis as well as the caregivers)
*Disagreements on what kind of help to get
* How to know where the Free or low-cost resources are in the community
*Knowing what you can do consistently that can help. The first action step to take.
*Thinking there is no light or hope in the darkness.
*You are thinking and feeling alone
*You think you deserve this because you have made mistakes that are beyond repair
*You are told by others that all you need is to pray longer and have more faith
*You are told you are evil
*Blame and Shame
*Stigma
*Treating the physical body and the mental symptoms separately that manifest (Example if you have a brain tumor you might manifest forgetfulness)
* Communication SKILLS Coming out of Silence

Balancing Justice and Mercy with Love and Rules
Enabling or allowing poor behavior
Using the diagnosis as a free pass for an excuse or poor behavior

SOLUTIONS
Mindfulness school
Community mental health website
Ask for ways to call in for ideas for reduced stress
Hotline for suicide
Journals
Family Stories-share successes and what you learned from failure
Know you are Loved no matter what you do or have done
Ask doctor if you can cut the pill in half to reduce cost
Scholarship Funding to help with insurance and medical costs
Jobs that will hire those with mental disabilities and know how to train them to be successful
Have a support base where they can go and make commitments and report back results
Use communication formula if acting in RED, Yellow or Green Zones

The worth of ONE is great! What matters to you, matters! You're not alone unless you choose to be!

Contribution-Care Giver
Mother with Loss of a Son

My son passed away at the age of 26. He ended his life after suffering with severe mental illness. He had been diagnosed with many mental and physical debilitating disorders: bi-polar, severe depression, extreme anxiety, borderline personality, ehlers danlos syndrome, paranoia, psychotic, Asperger's, schizophrenic and fiber myalgia. He also experienced opioid addiction. Towards the end of his life, he was in so much mental anguish and physical pain, there was no Doctor, Therapy, Psychiatrist, ECT treatment or ER that could ease his torment.

Now in hindsight, I can finally see this to be true, even after going over it in my head a million times as to what I could have done to change the outcome, as his Mother and caregiver. On a day to day basis, my husband and I would never know what each day would bring. We loved our son and tried desperately to be good caregivers. It seemed we were constantly fighting an uphill battle that could never be won.

Many times, my son would beg us for our help, and we would try to do all we could, then we would start to feel manipulated and then feel guilty for not meeting the endless needs of the "black hole" he felt inside, a black hole that could never be filled to what truly plagued him. Then there were the times we would back off, realizing we were trying too hard to rescue him and creating more problems. We wanted him to be self-reliant and safe and not depending on us for the rest of his life. With his mental and physical disabilities, we tried to teach him the skills and tools he would need to help him function on his own. Then often times it seemed his situation would go from bad to worse and we would step in and continue the cycle of rescuing.

As a caregiver, one of the hardest things for me was to watch my son suffer through the decisions he made or wouldn't make because of his disabling illness. If there was anything I could do to help, I would try to do it, but I had to learn the hard way that there is a fine line between healthy care giving and rescuing. Rescuing can be enabling. I have since learned that rescuing can often take away a person's agency to act for him or herself for opportunity to grow.

There were also those times when my spouse and I were not on the same page as to what would be best for our son and that usually led to marital stress and division and created a negative effect on the whole family including his other three siblings.

There were hopeful times, times when we would start to see the light at the end of the tunnel. Seeing our sweet, fun loving son start to take hold of his true potential and accomplish his goals; for he was very gifted. We wanted so much for him to be happy. I am so grateful for the good times we shared and I will always hold them dear in my heart.

Being a caregiver, I always did better when I was getting enough sleep and eating well, which I honestly did not do all the time, sometimes I let stress get the better of me. When I did take better care of myself, there was more of me to go around, and I could handle life a lot better and I might add, a little chocolate can go a long way too!

Writing a daily journal or log for my son was always helpful. I could go back to a certain day and see how he was doing behavioral wise or what medication might be affecting him. It helped a lot. There were times I needed "just me time" or time to get away with my husband or sisters. It made all the difference in the world!

In closing my contribution to this amazing and healing book, I would tell you (the reader) never give-up for the person you are care giving for. Even though my son is not here, I know his spirit has moved on. I am a Christian and I know that this world is not the end. I know I will see my son again and that brings a great deal of comfort and Joy to my soul. I know he is working on things there that he wasn't able to do here.

Contribution-
Mother's Perspective (Parent)

It was a pleasant surprise to read this book and discover tools to assist those who struggle with mental health issues and their caregivers who often travel this difficult journey with a loved one.

As a caregiver, I found an experience or two that might be helpful to others:

1- The loved one or patient can have super hearing. This actually can be used to help them.

For example I could whisper her name and say:

You are a wonderful person (pause) _____(her name)... you helped us today.

2-Tell Stories with descriptive phrases.

Another great tool that I found effective.

For example: (in a mild gentle tone)

You are walking on a beautiful sandy beach... Feel the soft squishy sand... Wiggle your toes... They are happy in the sand... The sun is warm on your face. ..Close your tired eyes and feel the warmth and rays sprinkle sunshine from your head to your toes... breath in and enjoy the gentle breeze...The light and warmth continues to shine upon you...

The narrative continues...

3-Do: Simple exercises

Example: jumping jacks or something like it to keep them busy. I found it to be very helpful and important to be mindful of energy levels on this journey together. Exercise can really help with this.

An example of this:

Ping-Pong

The loved one could certainly be out of it, but they still can actually do quite well. I could tell and it was quite evident when they got to the end of this activity because they would whack the ball until it would smash or crush the ball completely.

Amazingly enough, they can play this for quite a while and it's great exercise. Keeps them busy, safe, and out of trouble. (Again, not when they are in the red zone as it would not be good for them to have paddles or objects that could be thrown or cause damage or injury to themselves or others)

Different stages can go to different levels from maybe a whole day to just minutes. This is just the way it is. Understand that this is just the nature of the illness, so settle in and get used to it. That is not the same as giving up. Never give up. Love them always and forever.

4-Do: write a Journal

If they can write, (which sometimes they are not well enough to do), but if they can write it was something they can do to keep occupied and that is always a plus.

5-Sing Songs

This was more effective than just playing music because they are actively involved. Attention span is usually short and often requires change and adjustments to their needs (similar to dealing with a young kindergartner and about the same attention span). It is always a delight to find something that they like and respond well to.

By having them do simple tasks such as writing a journal or singing familiar sweet songs at times (if they can accept this). These activities can be very beneficial and effective. It can help keep them busy doing something calming and productive and allow the caregiver some welcome relief.

(Obviously this is not productive activities during the red zone)

In conclusion our daughter has learned likewise to keep herself as well and healthy as possible by using the resources that are available.

Our sweet daughter is beautiful and productive. She has always desired the best for others. Her husband is loyal and devoted to her. They are a shining example to many. It is a miracle that she is now an amazing author and has shared this message of illuminating love in the home, and consolidated these tender thoughts and feelings into this wonderful book. It was a very kind and personal gift to us. Full of challenges and hurdles, but with the idea that it can come as relief to many families suffering with trials and tribulations. Even if the only one is our own family that is the beneficiaries of this book, then it has been worth it. A very tall order, but worth it.

Love you dear daughter.

Contribution

Father's Perspective (Parent)

I would not want any comments that I make as a Father to detract from the beautiful message of both the content and message so beautifully expressed in this book, that of Illuminating Love In the Home. The truths and principles of the teachings of Jesus Christ have provided both strength and resolution to trials and troubled waters of life. These principles and truths when properly applied in the home are effective both in and out of the gospel of Jesus Christ. Love can and does heal both the body and the soul. Repeatedly Christ said in reference to the many miracles He performed that your faith hath made thee whole. As this book demonstrates faith without works is dead. We must work at and do the right things if we want our lives to be happy and fruitful. And it is well said that an ounce of prevention is worth a pound of cure. I am impressed with the suggested actions that you are encouraged to take to resolve or even prevent some of life's challenges,

*struggles, and mental illness and other trials we
may face.*

Beginning with one's self!

*My perspective as a Father is that I had a child
who all of her childhood, as well as adult life has
tried so very hard to be good. She has all too often
been extremely hard on herself. It was too easy as
a parent to overlook the need to help relieve her of
those inner apprehensions and self inflicted
wounds and guilt for incidents that were beyond
her control. I needed to have made her feel that
the door was always open to discuss whatever was
bothering her without reprisal. Knowing that no
matter what ... we love you. Perhaps in this as
parents we failed.*

*She held far to many of her feelings and troubles
to her self. Being the oldest child she was all too
often relied on to be the shining example to the
rest of the family and all too often was like a
second mother to her siblings, when in fact she
was just another child. There needed to have been
more loving communication between us. All too
often the needs of the moment took precedence*

over the consolation and understanding of the inner workings of the mind at any given time.

Having experienced a number of potential life threatening experiences in my life time, such as heart, cancer, saddle embolism, etc., I can say without reservation that mental illness is by far the most challenging experience that I have been through in this life. It is almost incomprehensible the feelings that a parent goes through watching a child change so radically from what they really are. That is the moment when true love needs to prevail and in time can be the healing balm that we all are looking for.

I am very proud and happy to see the beautiful person that my dear daughter really always was and has now become. I hope and wish that any one who reads the book will find joy and success as well as a personal resolution to whatever it is that ails them. As she has pointed out in her book the Love of God, Love of Yourself and the Love of those who Love You, along with the blessing of those who can help you find it, can bring happiness, joy, health and wellness to your life. Hopefully through application of these loving Christ like principles you will find it.